Basics of

Dental

Technology

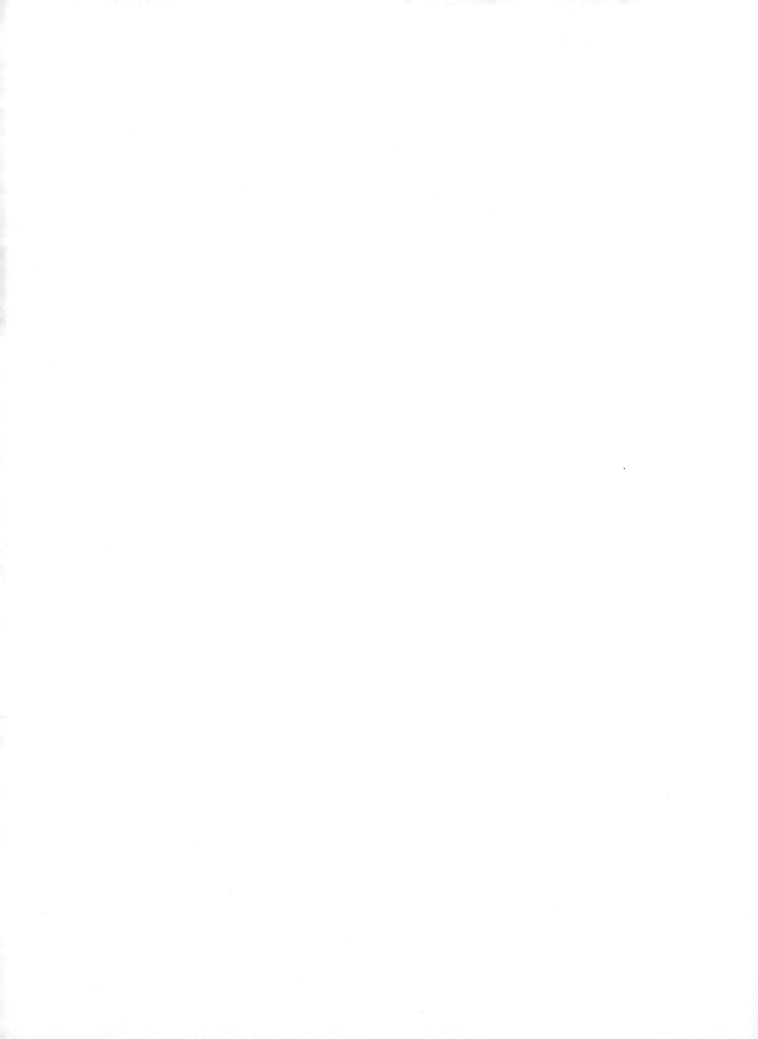

Basics of Dental Technology

A Step by Step Approach

Second edition

Tony Johnson
PhD, MMedSci, LCGI, MCGI, FETC, FHEA
Senior Lecturer
School of Clinical Dentistry
Academic Unit of Restorative Dentistry
University of Sheffield
UK

David G. Patrick
PhD, PgDip, FHEA
University Teacher
School of Clinical Dentistry
Academic Unit of Restorative Dentistry
University of Sheffield
UK

Christopher W. Stokes
BMedSci, PCHE, MEd, PhD, FHEA
Senior University Teacher
School of Clinical Dentistry
Academic Unit of Restorative Dentistry
University of Sheffield
UK

David G. Wildgoose
MPhil, LCGI, MCGI, FETC
Honorary Research Fellow
School of Clinical Dentistry
Academic Unit of Restorative Dentistry
University of Sheffield
UK

Duncan J. Wood
BMedSci, PhD, FHEA
Senior University Teacher
School of Clinical Dentistry
Academic Unit of Restorative Dentistry
University of Sheffield
UK

WILEY Blackwell

This edition first published 2016
© 2011, 2016 by John Wiley & Sons Ltd.

Registered office: John Wiley & Sons, Ltd, The Atrium, Southern Gate, Chichester, West Sussex, PO19 8SQ, UK

Editorial offices: 9600 Garsington Road, Oxford, OX4 2DQ, UK
The Atrium, Southern Gate, Chichester, West Sussex, PO19 8SQ, UK
1606 Golden Aspen Drive, Suites 103 and 104, Ames, Iowa 50010, USA

For details of our global editorial offices, for customer services and for information about how to apply for permission to reuse the copyright material in this book please see our website at www.wiley.com/wiley-blackwell

Library of Congress Cataloging-in-Publication Data

Johnson, Tony (Anthony Phillip), author.
Basics of dental technology : a step by step approach / Tony Johnson, David G. Patrick, Christopher W. Stokes, David G. Wildgoose, Duncan J. Wood. -- Second edition.
    p. ; cm.
    Includes index.
    Preceded by Basics of dental technology / Tony Johnson . . . [et al.]. 2011.
    ISBN 978-1-118-88621-2 (pbk.)   I. Patrick, David G., 1964- , author. II. Stokes, Christopher William, 1977- , author. III. Wildgoose, David G., author. IV. Wood, Duncan J., author. V. Title.
    [DNLM: 1. Technology, Dental--methods. 2. Technology, Dental--instrumentation. WU 150]
    RK652
    617.6′9--dc23
                                                                                        2015006395

A catalogue record for this book is available from the British Library.

Wiley also publishes its books in a variety of electronic formats. Some content that appears in print may not be available in electronic books.

Cover image: background image - © Batke/Getty Images

Set in 10/12pt Myriad Pro by SPi Global, Chennai, India
Printed and bound by CPI Group (UK) Ltd, Croydon, CR0 4YY

C9781118886212_120523

Contents

About the companion website

Basics of Dental Technology is accompanied by a companion website:

www.wiley.com/go/johnson/basicsdentaltechnology

The website includes:

- Multiple choice questions
- Downloadable images

Chapter 1 | INTRODUCTION

1.1 Introduction

This book has been designed for use in the dental laboratory as a guide for the novice dental technician. Described in the manner of a 'cook book', the procedures in this handbook have been designed to be followed step by step. Presented in sections ordered by specialty, each procedure has been completed in a dental laboratory, with photographs illustrating all the important steps of each procedure. The work shown in this book has not been edited or tweaked, but is presented as the instructions given in this book were followed, to ensure that the outcomes are achievable by anyone following the guides (perhaps with a little practice!).

1.2 How to use this book

Working impression ⟩ Casting working model ⟩ Sectioning

This book is designed for the student of dental technology for use on the bench in the dental laboratory. The construction of many dental prostheses and appliances requires progression through a series of stages, often from impression through to the finished product. You can use this book to work through each procedure step by step.

The graphic at the beginning of the sections will help you to see where any given procedure fits into the production process. An example of this is shown on the right.

For each procedure you will find a brief **introduction**, a list of the tools and **equipment required**, guidance on **working safely** and an illustrated step-by-step **basic procedure**.

In addition, the **hints and tips** sections give techniques to expand or refine the process, and the **extended information** sections give an insight into the scientific and clinical aspects that can enhance your understanding of the topic.

1.3 Equipment and instruments

The equipment listed below is commonly found in a dental laboratory, and with which any technician should be familiar.

Plaster bowl, spatula and knife (Figure 1.3.1)

Common to all plaster rooms, these items are used for mixing, shaping and trimming plaster of Paris, Kaffir and die stone materials. Cleanliness of these items is important to prevent rapid setting of materials.

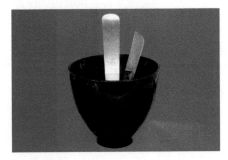

Figure 1.3.1

Basics of Dental Technology: A Step By Step Approach, Second Edition.
Tony Johnson, David G. Patrick, Christopher W. Stokes, David G. Wildgoose and Duncan J. Wood.
© 2016 John Wiley & Sons, Ltd. Published 2016 by John Wiley & Sons, Ltd.
Companion Website: www.wiley.com/go/johnson/basicsdentaltechnology

Wax knives and carvers

These instruments are commonly used in the laboratory for a number of procedures. You should purchase your own good-quality knives and carvers.

Small wax knife: Most commonly used in the fabrication of crowns for placing and carving inlay wax. You may see technicians using two, a cold and a hot knife, to save time (Figure 1.3.2, instrument on the left).

Large wax knife: Used for melting, placing and carving modelling wax in the production of dentures. Again, it is common to see two knives being used, a cold and a hot knife (Figure 1.3.2, instrument on the right).

LeCron carver: This carver is popular for the carving of inlay wax in the production of crowns. It is used cold, but some techniques use it slightly warm, but not hot (Figure 1.3.3, instrument on the far right).

Ash 5: This carver is used cold to shape modelling wax in the production of dentures (Figure 1.3.3, instrument in the centre).

Hylin carver: This carver is popular for the carving of inlay wax in the production of crowns. It is used cold (Figure 1.3.3, instrument on the far left).

PKT (PK Thomas): A set of instruments (examples of two shown) designed to aid the precise positioning of molten wax in the production of crowns (Figure 1.3.4).

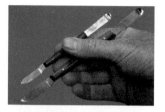

Figure 1.3.2

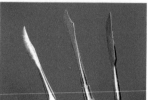

Figure 1.3.3

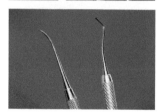

Figure 1.3.4

Other hand instruments

Ceramic brushes: Available in a range of sizes similarly to artists' brushes (Figure 1.3.5), with sizes from 0 to 20 with 0 being the smallest and 20 the largest. These brushes are made from sable and should be treated with care. A size 6 brush is popular for the placement of ceramics in the production of crowns. Smaller brushes are useful for staining, and a larger brush for condensing ceramic.

Ceramic spatulas: These instruments (Figure 1.3.6) are used for mixing, placing and carving of ceramic powders. They are produced from a material that will not contaminate the ceramic with metal particles that may cause discoloration.

Micromotors: Modern micromotors (Figure 1.3.7) are very advanced in terms of engineering, control and quality. They are powered by low voltage electricity and usually controlled via a foot or knee controller, allowing the speed to be set anywhere between 5000 and 40 000 rpm. The chuck is opened and closed by twisting the handpiece to secure or remove a bur.

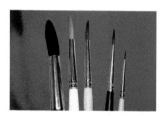

Figure 1.3.5

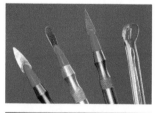

Figure 1.3.6

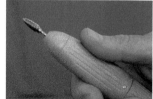

Figure 1.3.7

Burs

There is a huge range of burs currently on the market and manufacturers devote several pages of their catalogues to them. Below is a brief outline of the main types.

Tungsten carbide (TC): These are very popular burs used for many applications within the laboratory from trimming plaster to acrylic and metal. They are available in a large selection of shapes and sizes (Figure 1.3.8). The most useful are the plaster trimmers, flame-shaped for trimming acrylic and small round (often called rosehead) burs for accessing small areas.

Steel burs: As above, but not as hard wearing (and cheaper).

Stone burs: Abrasive stone burs are available in different grades, shapes, sizes and materials. The shapes range from cones to points to discs (Figure 1.3.9) and the different materials are indicated (often by colour) for different applications, that is, for the trimming and finishing of ceramics, acrylics or alloys.

Diamond discs and burs: Increasingly popular over the past decade, these tools are used for the shaping of ceramics and composites. They are available in many shapes and sizes (Figure 1.3.10).

Rubber abrasives for metals: These are available as wheels, cones or points and are used mainly in the finishing of metal surfaces (Figure 1.3.11).

Abrasives for acrylics: The simplest is a mandrel that holds a small piece of sandpaper, but rubber-bonded abrasives are now popular (Figure 1.3.12).

Brushes and mops: The main application of these is the polishing of metal surfaces in combination with wax-based polishing compounds (Figure 1.3.13).

Pliers and cutters

For orthodontic appliance manufacture (or for any other occasion where a wire may need to be bent or cut) the technician will have a selection of tools.

Adams 65: Square-ended pliers used in the bending of orthodontic stainless steel wire (Figure 1.3.14).

Adams 64: Square- and round-ended pliers used in the forming of springs and curves in orthodontic wires (Figure 1.3.15). (Sometimes referred to as 'half-round'.)

Maun cutters: Used for the cutting of orthodontic stainless steel wires (Figure 1.3.16).

Parallel pliers: Used for firmly griping a variety of items (Figure 1.3.17).

Large laboratory equipment

Most laboratories will have most or all of the following (illustrations of some of the following equipment will appear later in the book).

Model grinder: A bench-mounted, water-lubricated, tungsten carbide wheel used to grind plaster products (Figure 1.3.18).

Polishing lathe: Used with brushes and pumice, or mops and polishing wax in the polishing of acrylics and alloys (Figure 1.3.19). Modern lathes have integrated dust extraction and lighting and have two speeds: 1500 or 3000 rpm. The polishing

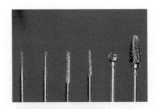

Figure 1.3.8

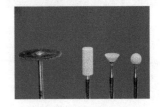

Figure 1.3.9

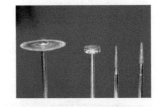

Figure 1.3.10

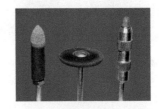

Figure 1.3.11

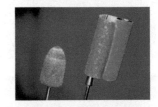

Figure 1.3.12

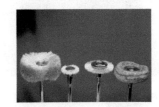

Figure 1.3.13

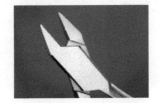

Figure 1.3.14

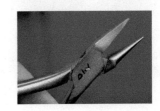

Figure 1.3.15

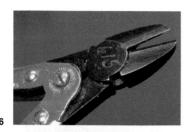

Figure 1.3.16

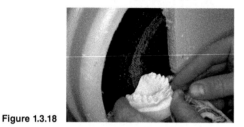

Figure 1.3.17

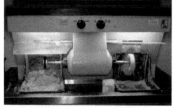

Figure 1.3.18

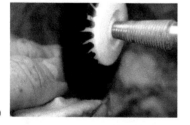

Figure 1.3.19

Figure 1.3.20

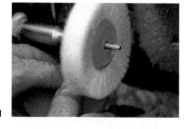

Figure 1.3.21

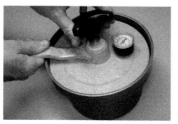

Figure 1.3.22

lathe can be fitted with a variety of brushes and mops, for example, a bristle brush for applying abrasive pumice to acrylics (Figure 1.3.20) or a cotton mop for polishing acrylics or alloys (Figure 1.3.21).

Steam cleaner: Used extensively in the dental laboratory for cleaning models and restorations.

Pressure bath: These use compressed air to keep self-curing acrylics under pressure during curing. They also have the facility to keep water warm to aid the process.

Hydroflask: Used full of water for putting self-curing acrylic under pressure whilst curing, in the repair of dentures, for example (Figure 1.3.22).

Vibrating table: Used during the mixing and pouring of plaster materials to help avoid air bubbles.

Vacuum mixer: Essential in the production of models for fixed prosthodontics and for mixing investment materials. This machine mixes plaster materials mechanically in a sealed pot whilst sucking the air out of the plaster mix.

Boiling out machine: This machine keeps water hot enough to remove wax from moulds (e.g. in the production of complete dentures). It has a compartment in which moulds can be placed and automatically sprayed, or often there is a hand-operated shower for manual spraying.

Presses: Presses are usually bench mounted and used to close denture flask (moulds). Hydraulic presses are also available for the same purpose. These work in the same way as a hydraulic car jack and require less force than manual presses.

Clamps: Denture flask clamps are used to keep flasks under pressure during the curing process required for heat-cured acrylics.

Denture flasks: Brass flasks used to create two-part moulds of wax trial dentures in the conversion to acrylic dentures.

Curing bath (dry heat or water): Used for the curing of heat-curing acrylic. Large enough to accept the mould and spring clamp, these machines have an automatic heating cycle to ensure optimum curing of the acrylic.

Porcelain furnace: These small, automated vacuum furnaces are specifically for the firing of ceramics (Figure 1.3.23). They are computerised and programmable, and can store the data for the various firing cycles required for different ceramics.

Burnout furnace: Relatively large for a dental technology laboratory, these furnaces are used in the heating of moulds and crucibles prior to casting. Modern furnaces are programmable to allow for preheating and the holding of high temperature during the heating cycle.

Casting machines: There are several types of casting machines combining the different casting forces (centrifugal, air pressure/vacuum) and different heating methods (induction, electrical resistance, gas torch, oxyacetylene).

High-speed grinder: Bench-mounted motor used with a cut-off disc or grinding wheel, for removing sprues and finishing cobalt–chromium alloy denture frameworks.

Spot welder: Used to weld stainless steel wire or components in the production of orthodontic appliances.

Ultrasonic bath: Used extensively for cleaning restorations or components of restorations in conjunction with different cleaning solutions.

Drying oven: A low temperature oven used for gently warming and drying refractory models used in the production of cobalt–chromium denture frameworks.

Electrolytic bath: Used in the 'polishing' of cobalt–chromium alloy frameworks.

Technician's workbench: The workbench is often fitted with drawers, a gas supply for Bunsen burners, electrical sockets, a micromotor, dust extraction and colour-balanced lighting.

Lighting: Lighting is an important feature of the dental laboratory in terms of long-term well-being for eyes working under demanding conditions. It is also essential to allow correct assessment of colour when producing aesthetic restorations. Tungsten or fluorescent lights can alter the perception of the shade being matched.

Shot-blaster: There are several types of shot-blaster using different sizes of abrasives (such as aluminium oxide or glass beads) for different purposes. Non-recirculating blasters are used in conjunction with extraction in the preparation and finishing of metal surfaces, for example, in the production of metal-ceramic restorations. Recirculating blasters are used with larger grit materials in the removal of investment materials from cobalt–chromium frameworks.

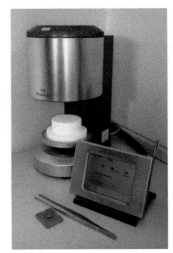

Figure 1.3.23

1.4 Health and safety in the dental laboratory

There are many hazards in the dental laboratory and many procedures that have an element of risk attached to them; however, if we take time to assess the risks and hazards, hopefully we will be able to minimise, or in some cases eliminate, the potential for harm.

It is the responsibility of all who work in the dental laboratory to ensure that we work safely and that we minimise the risk of injury to ourselves and others. It can be said that the effect of our use or misuse of equipment and materials can affect the degree of risk from known health hazards in the laboratory. In order to make sure that the working environment is a safe one there are some simple steps that can be taken, such as carrying out a 'risk assessment' and identifying any hazards present.

What are hazards?

A hazard is anything that could possibly be damaging.

What are risks?

How something might be damaging to you or others.

Risk assessment

A risk assessment is an examination of what could cause harm to people. A risk assessment is done so that one can decide whether enough precautions have been taken to prevent accidents or injury.

Workers and others have a right to be protected from harm caused by a failure to take reasonable control measures.

How to assess the risks in your workplace

The easiest and most effective way that you can assess the risks and put in place measures to minimise the risks in your workplace is to follow the five-step plan given below.

1. Identify all hazards

Walk around your workplace to see what may cause harm, check manufacturer's instructions on chemicals and think about long-term harm such as noise and dust.

2. Decide who might be harmed and how

Everyone does not have to be named, but specific groups of people have to be considered, such as plaster room workers or acrylic room workers; members of the public also need consideration if they have access.

3. Evaluate the risks and decide on the precautions

Once the risks have been identified, it has to be decided what can be done to minimise or eliminate the risk. This can be done by some simple means such as limiting access to hazardous chemicals or using less harmful chemicals and substances. Use protective clothing and organise work so that exposure is minimised.

4. Record all your findings and make sure to put them in practice

If proper notes are made it will be easier to implement safe working practices; also, remember to involve all staff so that a cohesive plan can be adopted by all to ensure the continued safety of all staff.

5. Regularly review your assessment and update when needed

All things are subject to change – number of employees, chemicals, working practices, etc. – so it is a good idea to review any risk assessment on at least a yearly basis so that any changes that have to be made can be done with relatively little disruption.

Assessing risks need not be an onerous task and if 'Risk Assessment' records are kept up to date, they can be carried out quickly and effectively with little hindrance to daily working practices.

Before starting to follow any procedure in this book, you should carry out a risk assessment. To help you, the **Working safely** section for each procedure outlines the main hazards.

1.5 Sterilisation and impression handling

Cross-infection in the dental laboratory

Cross-infection is a very real risk in the dental laboratory and one that should be taken seriously by all staff. Although it is the responsibility of the dentist to ensure that all items that are sent to the dental laboratory are sterilised, it is wise to treat everything with caution and not assume that we need not take basic precautions to minimise cross-infection.

The greatest risk to all members of the dental team is the patient and impressions that carry saliva; mucus and blood can pass disease on very easily. Workers in the dental laboratory do not usually see patients and in many cases are far away from the surgeries for which they carry out work. Being removed from the patient interface can lead to a feeling of not being directly involved with the clinical aspects of dentistry, but the impressions that we receive are a direct link with the patient and the clinic, and therefore must be treated accordingly.

Often the dentist will not know whether a patient has a communicable disease. Furthermore, the patient may not even know if they have a condition such as human immunodeficiency virus (HIV) infection or hepatitis so we have to make sure that we put into operation a cross-infection control procedure. Not only are we at risk from the patient but the patient also can be put at risk from the things that we do in the laboratory.

Cross-infection control procedure and policy

All laboratory staff should understand the cross-infection control procedure required in the dental laboratory and follow good practice.

(1) All staff involved in the production and preparation of dental models from impressions must be immunised against tetanus, hepatitis B, poliomyelitis, rubella, tuberculosis and diphtheria, and a record of their hepatitis B seroconversion must be held by the laboratory owner.

(2) The dental laboratory must provide personal protective equipment (PPE) for each laboratory worker, such as protective clothing, gloves, eyewear and masks that must be worn during all production procedures.

(3) All impressions and other items that have been in the patient's mouth or in contact with the patient/clinician/nurse, in any way, should have been sterilised and show evidence that they have been sterilised by the clinic sending them. They should be enclosed in a sealable plastic bag and have a sticker on them stating the date and time the sterilisation procedure was carried out.

(4) All areas handling impressions and dental casts must be cleaned with the appropriate disinfectant.

(5) In the event of a needlestick-type injury, the wound should be made to bleed, washed thoroughly under running water and covered with a waterproof dressing. The accident should be recorded in the accident book, and immediately advice sought from a qualified first aider as to whether any further action may be required.

(6) All potentially infected waste must be put in the correct bag. Appliances that are returned to the dental practice should be disinfected in a 1% solution of sodium hypochlorite for 10 minutes, rinsed under running water, and then packaged in a clean, single-use container within a 'clean area' of the laboratory.

(7) Eating and drinking is only permitted in designated areas.

(8) It is not the responsibility of the technician to sterilise any items of work leaving the dental laboratory. However, this should always be made clear to the clinic receiving the work, whose responsibility it is to sterilise any items of work before they enter the patient's mouth.

For further information contact the Dental Laboratories Association (DLA), British Dental Association (BDA), British Dental Trade Association (BDTA) or the Health & Safety Executive.

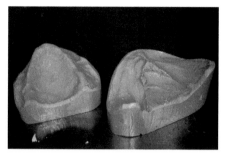

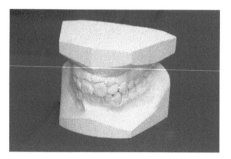

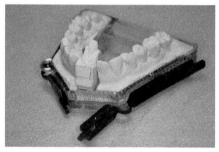

1.6 Introduction to model making

Most procedures in the dental laboratory are carried out on some form of plaster model, which is produced from an impression. There are several different model types that are produced for different applications.

In common to all is that care and attention to detail is required to produce an accurate, flaw-free model, which in turn will allow an accurate appliance, restoration, prosthesis or analysis to be made.

The types of model that will be discussed are the following:

- Models for prosthodontics (Figure 1.6.1)
- Orthodontic study models (Figure 1.6.2)
- Sectional models for indirect restorations (Figure 1.6.3).

Materials considerations

Dental models are almost always made from a plaster-based material. Before using these materials, it is important to have an understanding of their composition and handling characteristics.

Plaster of Paris

This is a type of building material based on calcium sulphate hemihydrate, and is often referred to as the 'beta form'. It is created by heating gypsum (the raw mineral) to about 150°C, which drives off the water to make the powder that is used in the dental laboratory. This powder is then mixed with water (typically 50 ml of water to 100 g of powder) to make a thick creamy mix suitable for dental applications.

Plaster of Paris is recognised in the dental laboratory as a white powder (other dental model materials are often coloured to differentiate them from it). The working time is about 3–4 minutes, and the initial set occurs after about 10 minutes. There is a slight expansion on setting in the order of 0.2–0.3%. The setting reaction is exothermic, so plaster of Paris models feel warm to the touch as they set. A rule of thumb to gauge if a model has set sufficiently to be handled is to check that it is cool to the touch (indicating that the setting reaction has completed).

Kaffir D

A more expensive gypsum-based, model-making material (and referred to as the 'alpha-form'), Kaffir D, has been heated in an autoclave (a sealed pressurised container) at around 130°C. The outcome is that more water is driven off and the powder produced is more regular in shape, finer and less porous. Less water is required to produce a mix suitable for dental model making (typically 20 ml of water to 100 g of powder), and the product is a significantly harder and stronger material.

Kaffir D is recognised in the dental laboratory by its yellow colour. The working time and setting time is usually slightly longer than normal plaster, but the expansion on setting is less at around 0.08–0.1%.

If it is used in equal parts with plaster of Paris, (referred to as a 50:50 mix), Kaffir D can be used for making edentulous models. A 50:50 mix results in a softer, weaker material than Kaffir D on its own, but harder and stronger than plaster of Paris. When making dentate models, a higher strength is required and Kaffir D should be used on its own.

Class IV die stone

This is the strongest, hardest and most accurate gypsum-based model material used in the laboratory. Sometimes called artificial stone, die stone, densite, improved stone or 'alpha-modified', it is formed by boiling gypsum in a 30% aqueous solution of calcium chloride and magnesium chloride. This process produces the smoothest, most compact particles of the three types described here.

A mix suitable for dental model making is typically 20 ml of water to 100 g of powder (although you should check the manufacturer's instructions), and the product is a significantly harder and stronger material. Care should be taken when mixing these materials to ensure that the optimum strength and accuracy is achieved. This is the only one of the three materials described here that is regularly mechanically mixed under vacuum.

Manufacturers often colour Class IV die stone (many different colours are used) to help distinguish it from plaster of Paris and Kaffir D. The working time and setting time is the longest of the three materials described here, with a working time of about 5 minutes, and a setting time of 20 minutes. The expansion on setting is around 0.05–0.07%.

Class IV die stone materials are used whenever a very strong and abrasion-resistant model is required or where the model may need to be sectioned, such as most crown and bridge work and constructing some cast metal partial denture frameworks.

Notes on mixing

With each of the materials above, changes in the powder to water ratio will affect the working and setting times, material strength and hardness and setting expansion.

As a rule of thumb, by using more water the setting time is extended, but the strength of the set material is reduced. Increasing the mixing time will reduce the setting time, but will tend to increase the setting expansion.

Additives, such as sodium chloride (table salt) and other 'setting solutions', act to significantly increase the setting time of a plaster mix, and can be useful when a fast set is required (such as for plaster impressions and articulating models).

1.7 Models for prosthodontics – casting primary impressions

Primary impression taking   Primary impression casting   Customised tray construction

Accurate impression taking and model making are essential to the successful production of a prosthetic device. If either procedure is carried out poorly, the appliance constructed on the model will not accurately fit the patient's mouth.

Primary impressions are taken in 'stock trays', which are ready-made trays. These are available in a range of sizes; however, they rarely fit the patient's mouth perfectly. The poor fit results in inaccuracies that are discussed further in the

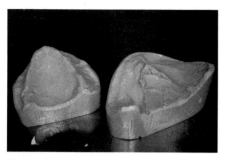

Figure 1.7.1

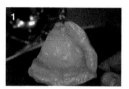
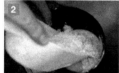
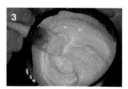
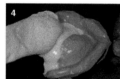
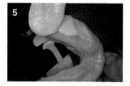
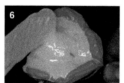
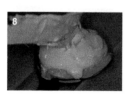
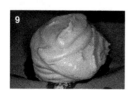
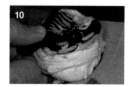

Extended information section below. To overcome these inaccuracies, a 'customised tray' is constructed (see Chapter 2), which is tailor-made for the patient on the primary model (Figure 1.7.1).

You will need:

- Gloves
- Plaster of Paris/dental stone (Kaffir D)
- Plaster bowl, spatula and knife
- Weighing scales
- Measuring cylinder
- Vibrating table
- Model trimmer
- Indelible pencil

Basic procedure

1. Rinse the impression under the tap to remove any remaining disinfectant, tissue or napkin. Shake off the excess water.

2. For each impression add approximately 120 ml of water to a plaster bowl. To this, add approximately 300 g of powder in a 50:50 ratio of plaster of Paris and dental stone (Kaffir D).

3. Mix with a spatula, avoiding air bubbles being trapped in the mixture until all lumps of powder are crushed and incorporated and a smooth consistency is achieved.

4. For the upper impression, place a small amount of the mixture onto the palate of the upper impression and hold firmly against a vibrating table or hand vibrate against the side of the mixing bowl to allow the material to fill the surface detail.

5. For the lower impression, add to the retromolar pad region on one side only and vibrate the mix into the impression.

6. Do not allow the model material to flow quickly over the impression; instead produce a wash of material. Air trapped between the model material and the impression will cause voids in the model surface.

7. Extra care should be taken with partial denture impressions, as it is essential that the material fills each tooth. Using a fine bristle brush to encourage the mix into the tooth areas is a useful technique.

8. Add material until the impression is full, leaving a slightly domed top.

9. Form a base on the bench approximately the diameter of the impression and 30 mm deep. Now wash your bowl and spatula.

10. Invert the impression on to the base once it is capable of supporting the weight of the impression, just before the initial set. The impression tray should be parallel to the bench top and the base should be approximately 25 mm high.

Continued over

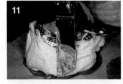
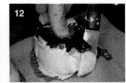
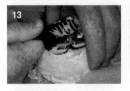
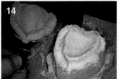

11. When the material has set such that the excess can be removed without disturbing the remainder, remove the excess material from around the impression using a plaster knife. Ensure that the area between the tray and the bench are full.

12. To ensure easy removal of the impression from the model, the plaster should extend 2–3 mm on to the impression, but should not extend onto the metal or plastic impression tray.

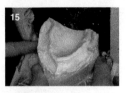

13. After 30 minutes the impression should be removed. Remove any plaster locking the tray on to the model with a plaster knife. Hold the base of the model to the bench top with one hand and pull the impression up vertically using the handle. For dentate models, remove along the long axis of the incisor teeth.

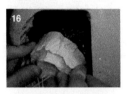

14. Put the impressions to one side.

15. Using the model trimmer, trim the back of the models such that the midline of the model is at right angles to it.

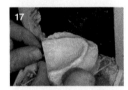
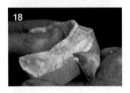

16. Stand the model on this edge and reduce the thickness of the base until flat and parallel to the alveolar bone or occlusal plane. Do not reduce the thickness to such an extent that the palate or sulcus is perforated.

17. Trim the periphery of the model by placing on the flat base, leaving a 'land area' of 2–3 mm around. This protects the impression surface and allows the user to differentiate between the impression and the side of the model.

18. Clean up the edges using a plaster knife, being careful not to scratch the model.

19. After drying, label the models using an indelible pencil.

Extended information

Inherent problems with primary impressions are as follows:

- Over-extension: Over-extensions of the buccal sulcus are due to the use of excessive impression material. This material is displaced into the sulcus during impression taking and pushes the cheeks out, creating a false record of the sulcus.

- Distortion: As the impression tray does not fit well, the impression material is not uniform in thickness. This causes distortion due to the material contracting on setting and during storage. Where the material is thin, only a small amount of contraction will occur, but where there is increased thickness, larger amounts will occur leading to distortion.

Continued over

Hints and tips

- Use a clean bowl and spatula. Contaminants will cause the plaster to set more quickly.
- Do not over-mix the material, as this will also cause it to set more quickly.
- Mixing under vacuum is the most effective method of achieving a smooth, air-free mixture.

- Lack of surface detail: The material used for primary impressions is usually mixed to have a relatively high viscosity in order that it remains within the impression tray. For recording surface detail, a low-viscosity material is required.

To overcome these problems whilst working, or secondary, impressions are taken using a customised or 'special' tray.

1.8 Models for prosthodontics – boxing-in impressions

The method described in Section 1.7 for casting primary impressions could be criticised on two counts. Firstly, that on inverting the impression onto the plaster base, distortion of the impression material may occur if the base plaster is too firm, particularly if unsupported impression material is present. Secondly, as the plaster sets, the water in the mixture will rise, creating a weaker material at the surface of the model.

To overcome these potential faults, the impressions to be cast may be 'boxed-in' (Figure 1.8.1) and the model poured such that the fitting surface of the model is at the bottom of the model (inverted) during setting. The disadvantage with this method is the increase in working time and potential damage to the impression periphery during the wax attachment to the impression.

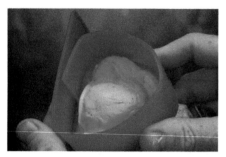

Figure 1.8.1

Work safety

Protective gloves should always be worn when handling impressions; refer to Section 1.5 on sterilisation and impression handling. Inhalation of plaster powder should be avoided.

You will need:

- Gloves
- Plaster of Paris/dental stone (Kaffir D)
- Plaster bowl, spatula and knife
- Weighing scales
- Measuring cylinder
- Vibrating table
- Model trimmer
- Indelible pencil
- Soft wax strips
- Boxing-in wax sheets
- Bunsen burner

Basic procedure

1. Position soft wax strips around the periphery of the impression to leave about 3 mm of the sulcus showing. Seal to the impression with molten wax.

2. Wrap the sheet wax around the wax strip to form a box (you will need to fill in the centre of lower impressions with additional wax).

3. Mix the model material as described in Section 1.7 and carefully pour into the impression. The plaster will settle on the impression surface and water will rise to the top.

4. After setting, remove the wax and trim and finish the model as described in Section 1.7.

1.9 Models for prosthodontics – casting working (secondary) impressions

Secondary impression taking ▸ Secondary impression casting ▸ Registration rims production

A working model is produced from the working (or secondary) impressions. These are easily identified in the laboratory as the impressions will have been taken in a customized impression tray. The working model will form the basis of any future prosthesis, and so is cast with additional care, and from a stronger plaster mix to reduce the risk of damage or abrasion.

With the following exceptions, the casting of working impressions is identical to the casting of primary impressions.

You will need:
- Equipment list from Section 1.7
- Permanent felt-tipped pen

Work safety
Protective gloves should always be worn when handling impressions; refer to Section **1.5** on sterilisation and impression handling. Inhalation of plaster powder should be avoided.

Basic procedure

1. Use a permanent felt-tipped pen to mark a line around the periphery of the impression about 3 mm up the buccal reflection of the cheeks. This ensures that the final model will be complete.

2. When the cast impression is turned over onto the plaster base, allow the plaster to rise up the outer wall of the impression to the felt-tipped pen mark. This will provide a reflection of the sulcus on the model and allow a land area of 2–3 mm width to be formed.

3. Cast the model in 75:25 stone/plaster mixture to increase the hardness of the material and provide better abrasion resistance. This will minimise the damage caused when forces are applied during denture construction and processing of the acrylic resin.

4. The cast impression should be left to set for at least 45 minutes prior to removal of the impression.

5. Zinc-oxide/eugenol impression material will require softening in hot water before the trays can be removed.

6. The trays should be loosened all round the model and then removed slightly anteriorly in a vertical direction from the model without twisting. Twisting could cause damage to the model.

7. The finished model is trimmed to provide 2–3 mm of land area and a 1–3 mm reflected sulcus.

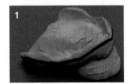

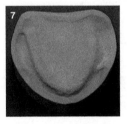

1.10 Models for prosthodontics – models for cobalt–chromium frameworks

Secondary impression taking ▸ Secondary impression casting ▸ Metal framework production

Working models for cobalt–chromium or other metal partial denture bases should be cast using Class IV die stone. This gives the model increased strength and abrasion resistance, which is needed to withstand the frequent placement and removal of the metal base during construction.

Apart from the description above, the casting of models for cobalt–chromium denture bases is the same as previously described for 'casting primary impressions' (Section 1.7).

You will need:

- Equipment list from Section 1.7
- Vacuum mixer and mixing pot
- Replace dental stone with Class IV die stone

Hints and tips

Removal of the impression may cause damage to lone-standing teeth. Where vulnerable teeth exist it may be necessary to section the custom-made impression tray with a cut-off disc to allow safe removal of the impression.

Basic procedure

Cast the impression as for working models (Section 1.7) with the following exceptions:

1. Class IV die stone should be vacuum mixed.

2. Class IV die stone should be left for at least 4 hours to set.

Impression casting ▷ Appliance design ▷ Component construction

1.11 Orthodontic study models

You will need:

- Orthodontic stone (white)
- Orthodontic model trimmer or three set squares: 20°, 39° and 60°
- Orthodontic model base-formers
- Plaster knife and spatula
- Vacuum mixing machine and mixing pot (100 g per model)
- 600-grit glass paper

Study models are used to provide information of a patient's occlusion. Orthodontic study models are produced such that the angulation of their exterior surfaces does not suggest any abnormalities or malalignment of the teeth. The bases are trimmed symmetrically about the midline to aid the eye in judging the symmetry of the dental arches. This trimming of the models also allows them to stand in the correct occlusal relationship and makes them easier to handle and store.

There are two methods of producing study models:

One-stage method: The impression is poured and inverted onto on to the base and trimmed as described previously. A mould may be used to form the angles of the base.

Two-stage method: Models are cast that are a minimal size, referred to as rims, and then set into bases at a later date.

Basic procedure

1. Clean the impression trays and check whether the impression is central within the impression tray. If not, mark the centre line on the impression to aid placement. Rinse the impressions under running water.

2. Vacuum mix the stone to a stiff consistency for 30 seconds to eliminate air bubbles.

Continued over

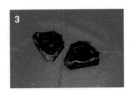

3. Fill the moulds with stone or make a base on the bench top.

4. Place a small amount of stone on the posterior border of the impression and let it flow to the anterior teeth whilst holding the impression on the edge of a vibrating table.

5. Remove the stone by tapping the impression on the side of the mixing bowl. This should leave a light covering of stone within the impression and help eliminate any air holes in the finished model.

6. Refill the impression as before and place to rest ready for inverting.

7. Invert the impression onto the moulds, keep the bottom of the tray level with the bench surface and centre the impression over the mould and check the midline position.

8. Trim excess plaster away from around the mould and leave to set.

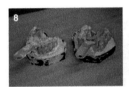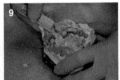

9. The trays should be loosened all round the model and then removed slightly anteriorly in a vertical direction from the model without twisting. Twisting could damage the model.

10. Check the models thoroughly for flaws.

11. Remove the base moulds.

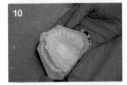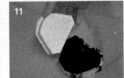

12. Firstly, make sure that the upper and lower models can be occluded without the wax bite, then make sure that the wax bite fits – be careful not to damage the incisors. The wax bite for study models should not cover the incisors; if it does, trim it off.

Model trimmers have built-in aids to enable the bases to be trimmed to the desired angles. The midline of the upper palate is used to assess the symmetry of the upper arch and as a reference to which the angles of the bases are cut.

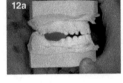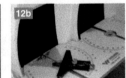

13. Using the model trimmer, trim the bases of the upper and lower models until parallel.

14. Trim the back edge of the upper model so that the midline of the model is at right angles to it.

15. Place the models in occlusion using the wax bite, and trim the back edge of the lower model to match the upper.

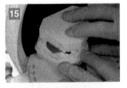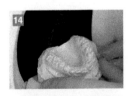

16. Set the angle on the platform of the model trimmer to 70°. With the models in occlusion, place the back edge of one model against the guide on the platform and trim the buccal side of the models until the sulcus is reached. Repeat for the other side.

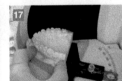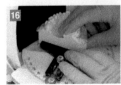

17. Repeat step 17 for the other side.

Continued over

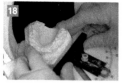
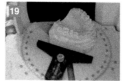
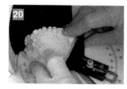
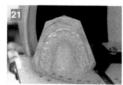
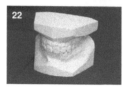

18. Set the angle guide to 25°. Trim the distal corner by placing the trimmed buccal surface against the guide.

19. Repeat step 19 for the other side.

20. With the angle still at 25°, trim the anterior surfaces to form a point at the midline by placing the back edge in contact with the angle guide.

21. Trim the front edge of the other model to follow the line of the arch.

22. The finished models can be given a final polish with sandpaper if required.

Hints and tips

Bases should be symmetrical with:

- Anterior surfaces finishing approximately at the canine
- Buccal surfaces finishing at the distal of the last molar
- Distal surfaces should end about midway across the last molar.

The lower model base should be approximately one-third thicker than that of the upper.

Study models can be finished with fine sandpaper to produce a smooth finish free from marks left by the model trimmer.

Extended information

Study models are used in orthodontics for three main reasons:

1. To provide a three-dimensional record of a patient's occlusion

2. To assess the position of the teeth in relation to the midline, allowing the amount of drift and symmetry to be monitored

3. To see progress in treatment.

Orthodontic study models are generally poured in white dental stone rather than plaster of Paris. Stone is preferred due to its hardness, durability and stability over a long period of time. Impressions are taken in alginate and therefore care must be taken to avoid loss of integrity.

The impression should be poured as soon as possible to retain its integrity and to avoid syneresis. This is where gel molecules in alginate are drawn closer together and as a result fluid exudates appear at the surface, which will result in poor surface quality.

At one time it was recommended that the base of the upper model should be trimmed so that its top surface corresponded with the Frankfort plane, resulting in rather tall and bulky models. The use of cephalometrics in relating the teeth and occlusion to the face and head has resulted in this being unnecessary.

Working impression ▷ Casting working model ▷ Sectioning ▷

1.12 Introduction to sectional models

Sectional models allow parts of the model to be removed independently and replaced accurately. Models for indirect fixed restorations are made in this way to allow each prepared tooth to be an individual section. There are two types of sectional models: tray systems and pinned systems.

Pinned systems are considered more accurate and are indicated where multiple dies are being used on the same model, for example, where a bridge is being constructed and accuracy is essential. Tray systems are easier and quicker to produce and are sufficiently accurate for simple cases.

Prior to casting a sectional working model, check:

- The type of impression material that has been used
- That the stock tray is rigid or the custom tray is well designed.

When checking the quality of the impression, common problems are:

- Impression material becoming unstuck from the tray
- Incorrect relocation of impression where a two-stage technique is used
- Teeth contacting the tray through the impression material
- Incomplete mixing of material (looks streaky and has tacky surface)
- Contaminants such as saliva
- Air voids in areas requiring accuracy
- Drags – which appear as elongated areas due to the removal of impression prior to setting
- Incomplete surfaces owing to insufficient material or premature setting
- Incomplete arch, when a complete arch is required.

1.13 Producing a sectional model using a tray system (Figure 1.13.1)

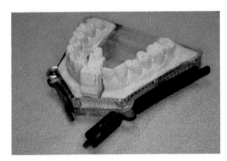

Figure 1.13.1

You will need:

- A good-quality impression (see Section 1.12)
- Prescription card
- Permanent marker
- Scalpel
- Surface tension relieving agent
- One tray base with retention lugs or pins
- Boxing-in wax
- Class IV die stone (100 g per model)
- Water
- Plaster knife and spatula
- Vacuum mixing facilities (including pot)
- Vibrating table
- Plaster bur
- Steam cleaner

Work safety

Care should be taken when handling the die stone powder as inhalation can be dangerous. Observe warnings on the surface tension reducing agent. Protective gloves should always be worn when handling impressions.

Basic procedure

1. Trim the periphery of the impression to the height of the top of the impression tray or to 3–5 mm above the gingival margin, whichever is highest.

2. Trim the palate of the impression to the same height as the periphery if not required for the treatment plan.

Continued over

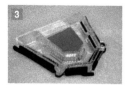

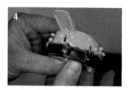

3. Prepare the tray by inserting the retention lugs and palatal block-out plate where required.

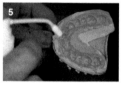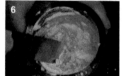

4. Looking through the base of the tray, position the impression such that the teeth are in the centre of the horseshoe-shaped trough. Record this position by making three marks with a permanent marker.

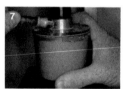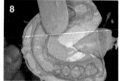

5. Spray the impression material with a surface tension reducing agent. Gently blow off the excess agent from the impression using an air line until dry.

6. Weigh the die stone powder into a dry mixing pot (typically 100 g). Add water (typically 20 ml) to the pot and hand mix briefly to incorporate the powder into the water.

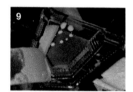

7. Vacuum mix for approximately 40 seconds.

8. With the impression on the vibrating table, pour the mixed die stone into the impression. To avoid air bubbles, start from the distal of one side and slowly fill the impression by chasing the die stone around. Make sure you see the material fill each tooth in turn. If in doubt, pour out and refill.

9. Fill the tray base level with the top. Add any remaining mixture to the top of the impression.

10. Wash the pot and stirrer whilst the material is fluid.

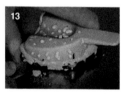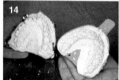

11. Turn the impression onto the base once the shine on the surface of the die stone has dulled (the die stone is beginning to set). You will need to check periodically for this.

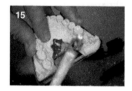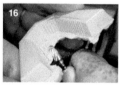

12. Using a plaster knife, remove any excess material from around the tray and impression. Leave to set for at least 60 minutes.

13. Remove any die stone preventing removal of the impression from the base using a plaster knife.

14. Remove the impression by gently easing vertically in line with the long axis of the teeth. Use a plaster knife to gently lever the tray if removal is difficult.

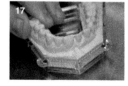

15. Remove the model from the tray. First remove the tray retention lugs, and then tap on the base of the tray (gently) to release the model.

16. Trim the excess die stone to neaten the model using a plaster trimming bur.

17. The periphery of the tray base should be seen clearly.

18. Clean all parts using the steam cleaner to finish.

1.14 Producing a sectional model using a pinned system

There are numerous types of pins available; these differ in material and anti-rotational design. Pinned systems take longer to produce but are more accurate.

You will need:

- A good-quality impression (see below)
- Prescription card
- Permanent marker
- Scalpel
- Surface tension relieving agent
- Model pins (and sleeves if required)
- Model drill system
- Cyanoacrylate glue
- Boxing-in wax

- Class IV die stone (100 g per model)
- Water
- Plaster knife and spatula
- Vacuum mixing facilities (including pot)
- Vibrating table
- Plaster bur
- Steam cleaner
- Plaster-separating solution

Work safety

Care should be taken when handling the die stone powder as inhalation can be dangerous. Observe warnings on the surface tension reducing agent. Protective gloves should always be worn when handling impressions.

Basic procedure

1. Trim the periphery of the impression to the height of the top of the impression tray or to 3–5 mm above the gingival margin, whichever is higher.

2. Trim the palate of the impression to the same height as the periphery if not required for the treatment plan.

3. Spray the impression material with surface tension reducing agent.

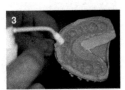

4. Gently blow off the excess surface tension reducing agent from the impression using an air line until dry.

5. Weigh the die stone powder into a dry mixing pot (typically 100 g).

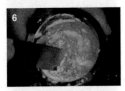

6. Add the water (typically 20 ml) to the pot and hand mix briefly to incorporate the powder into the water.

7. Vacuum mix for approximately 40 seconds.

8. With the impression on the vibrating table, pour the mixed die stone into the impression. To avoid air bubbles, start from the distal of one side and slowly fill the impression by chasing the die stone around. Make sure you see the material fill each tooth in turn. If in doubt, empty and refill.

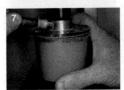
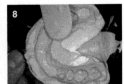

9. Wash the pot and stirrer whilst the material is fluid.

Continued over

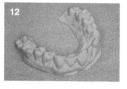
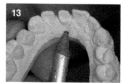
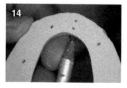
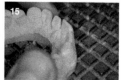
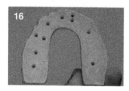
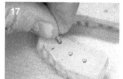
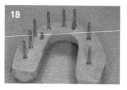
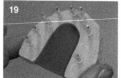
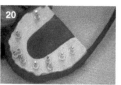
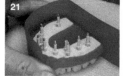
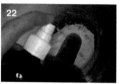
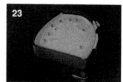
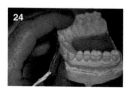
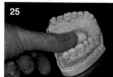
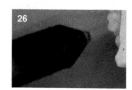

10. Leave the impression to set, tray-side down, for at least 60 minutes.

11. Using a plaster knife, remove the horseshoe-shaped model by gently easing vertically in line with the long axis of the teeth.

12. Trim the base of the model on the model trimmer to create a flat base.

13. You need to identify the teeth that are going to be worked on, as these will require two pins (or a double pin) to stop it rotating once sectioned.

14. The remaining sections of the model should also have more than one pin to stop rotation.

15. Drill two holes per section using a model drilling machine.

16. Check that the holes are located well within the edges of the model (as shown).

17. Fix the pins to the drilled holes using glue.

18. If required, place sleeves on each pin.

19. Block out the palate using boxing-in wax.

20. Place two layers of beading wax around the periphery of the model.

21. With the occlusal surfaces on the bench top, create a box using sheet wax high enough to cover the pins.

22. Spray the base of the die stone with plaster-separating solution.

23. Fill the boxed-out area with a mix of 50:50 plaster and Kaffir D to the top of the sleeves.

24. Allow the new base to set for at least 20 minutes. Remove the bulk of wax and place the model in hot water both to remove excess wax and to use the mismatch in thermal expansion of the die stone to the Kaffir D to help the two parts of the model separate.

25. Separate the two parts by pressing down in the centre of the palate.

26. Steam clean the model to finish.

Casting Working Model › Sectioning › Ditching

1.15 Sectioning the model

Sectioning allows removal of dies or parts of the model as required for restoration production (Figure 1.15.1). Parallel saw cuts are made through the model to enable removal of sections.

Ideally, the model should be completely dry before sectioning (at least 12 hours should have elapsed since casting).

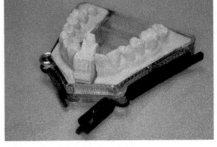

Figure 1.15.1

You will need:

- Dry die stone model (see Sections 1.13 and 1.14)
- Fret saw
- Plaster bur
- Pencil

Work safety

Use dust extraction when cutting and trimming the die stone.

Basic procedure

1. Pinned models can be sectioned whole, but tray system models should be removed from the tray base by removing the retaining lugs.

2. Mark the ideal cutting lines with a pencil. These should be parallel.

3. Place the saw blade on the plaster and carefully start the saw cut, avoiding both the margin and the adjacent teeth. Keep the cut straight and following the pencil line. If the saw cut deviates, it may be necessary to cut from the bottom up.

4. Repeat for each cut required.

5. Tidy the saw cuts with a bur and clean all components with the steam cleaner. Ensure tray base locating grooves are free from debris.

6. Refit all components and ensure that the die can be removed independently of the adjacent sections.

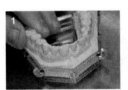
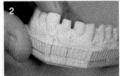
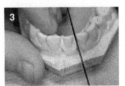
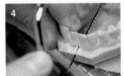
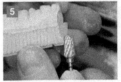
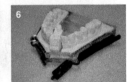

Hints and tips

When using a fret saw, apply very light pressure, using long saw strokes.

Extended information

Class IV die stones are commonly used for the production of sectional models due to the ease of use and relative cost. Other materials in use are:

- Scannable die stones: indicated for some CAD-CAM production routes

- Epoxy resins

- Copper plating

1.16 Introduction to articulating models

Articulators are mechanical devices that reproduce the movements of the mandible. Models are mounted on the articulator to allow the teeth to be seen in function. Simple hinge articulators are also available that hold models in intercuspal position (ICP).

To reproduce the movements accurately the models must be positioned at the correct distance from the condyle (hinge of the jaw). There are two methods of achieving this. The first is to use an **average** relationship between the teeth and the condyle, the second is to use a facebow to mechanically record this relationship on the patient and use this recording to position the models on the articulator.

Occlusal registration records

For dentate patients, the models may be mounted with or without an occlusal registration record. If the teeth interdigitate (mesh) well and it is clear that the models will be easy to relate, then no record will be used. However, if there is little interdigitation of the teeth, the clinician will send an occlusal registration to aid the technician in locating the models together. Registrations may be taken in wax, silicone or impression plaster.

For partially dentate patients, the clinician may use a partial registration rim to fill the edentulous areas and stabilise the models during the mounting procedure.

For edentulous patients, wax registration rims are produced, which are used in the mouth to record the necessary information: occlusal plane, centre line, position of teeth, vertical dimension and centric relation.

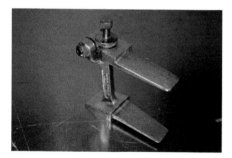

Figure 1.17.1

1.17 Articulating models on a simple hinge articulator

Simple hinge articulators (Figure 1.17.1) are limited in their range of use because they are unable to mimic the mandibular movements. However, the articulator is useful for holding study models together, holding models during the manufacture of simple appliances and for maintaining the vertical dimension during relining or repairing a denture.

Work safety

Care should be taken when using the model trimmer to ensure that your fingers or any other part of your body or clothing does not come into contact with the wheel. Eye protection should be worn at all times when using the model trimmer.

You will need:

- Models
- Registration blocks (edentulous) *or* occlusal registration (dentate)
- Simple hinge articulator
- Model trimmer
- Plaster of Paris
- Plaster bowl, spatula and knife
- Sticky wax

Basic procedure

1. Ensure the models are firmly fixed together in the correct occlusion.

2. Make sure the simple hinge articulator is adjusted to have enough room between the two arms to accommodate the two models; lightly apply Vaseline to the arms.

3. Mix plaster of Paris and form a pile on a piece of paper of the diameter of the mandibular model and between 10 and 20 mm high.

4. Embed the lower arm of the articulator into the centre of the plaster pile and press down until the foot of the articulator sits on the bench.

5. Add more of the plaster to the pile to cover the arm of the articulator.

6. Seat the mandibular model onto the pile of plaster and position so that the occlusal plane is level with the bench and the two models fit between the two arms of the articulator.

7. Place plaster of Paris on the top of the maxillary model and then close down the upper arm of the articulator onto the pile of plaster.

8. Place more plaster around the upper arm of the articulator until it is well covered.

9. The plaster of Paris can then be trimmed and tidied with a plaster knife.

10. Wait for at least 20 minutes for the plaster to set.

11. Once the plaster has fully set, the models can be separated, removed from the two arms of the articulator and the mounting plaster and finished by grinding smooth on a model trimmer.

12. A final smooth finish can be applied by sandpapering.

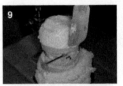
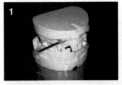
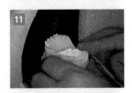
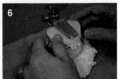
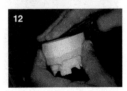
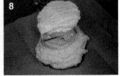
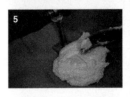
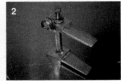
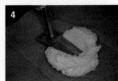
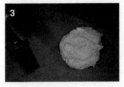
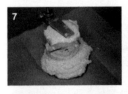
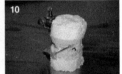

1.18 Articulating dentate models using the average position

The split-cast mounting technique allows the models to remain firmly in place for setting up the teeth, but permits them to be removed from their mountings and replaced later should further occlusal adjustment be required.

Work safety

Care should be taken when using the model trimmer to ensure that your fingers, or any other part of your body or clothing, does not come into contact with the wheel. Eye protection should be worn at all times when using the model trimmer.

You will need:

- Models
- Occlusal registration
- Average-value articulator
- Model trimmer
- Plaster of Paris
- Elastic band
- Plaster bowl, spatula and knife
- Sticky wax
- Modelling clay

1. Set the articulator's incisal pin to its 0° position and lock the condyles into the hinging position. Position the mounting plates or nuts as required.

2. Remove any artefacts that are a result of air blows from the occlusal surfaces of the teeth and trim the occlusal registration (bite registration) to the cusps of the teeth such that the fit may be assessed. Check that it fits accurately on to each model independently and when the models are arranged together. Double check that the heels of the models do not interfere.

3. Secure the models and registration to each other using sticky wax.

4. Trim the sides of the models to a taper (approximately 20°) along the front, sides, back and corners, using the model trimmer. Alternatively, cut grooves into the base of the models. This allows the models to be repositioned if removed (split-cast mounting technique).

5. Use three mounds of modelling clay on the lower arm of the articulator to support the models on the articulator. Adjust the position of the models to conform to the Bonwill triangle.

   Bonwill triangle: A 102-mm equilateral triangle formed from lines joining the condyle heads with the mesio-incisal angles of the lower central incisors (not always possible, so the uppers can be used instead).

6. The lower lateral incisors just contact the incisal indicator pin.

7. The occlusal plane corresponds to an elastic band placed around the articulator and into the notches provided.

8. Coat the top and tapered sides of the maxillary model with plaster-separating solution.

9. With the articulator open, mix plaster and place on the upper model trying to create a tall mound – this will avoid plaster spilling over the sides of the model.

10. Place the plaster onto and around the mounting plate on the articulator.

11. Whilst the plaster is still soft, close the articulator gently and ensure that the incisal pin is contacting the table.

12. Use a plaster knife to fill any remaining gaps between the articulator and model. The plaster will be neatened on the model trimmer later.

13. Allow to set for at least 10 minutes.

14. Turn the articulator upside down and remove the modelling clay.

Continued over

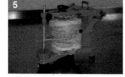
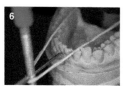
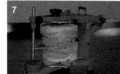
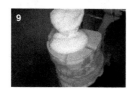
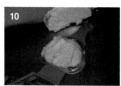
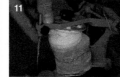
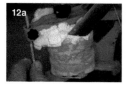
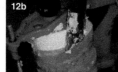

15. Apply the plaster-separating solution; then mix plaster and place on the lower articulating plate.

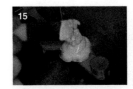

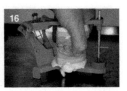

16. Gently close the articulator until the incisal pin touches the table.

17. Use a plaster knife to fill any remaining gaps between the articulator and model. The plaster will be neatened on the model trimmer later.

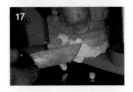

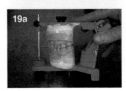

18. When set, the mounting plaster and models can be removed from the articulator and trimmed smooth on the model trimmer.

19. Replace the mounted models back onto the articulator and ensure that the incisal pin touches the table and that the models occlude correctly.

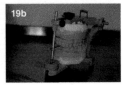

1.19 Articulating edentulous models using the average position

You will need:

- Models
- Registration blocks
- Average-value articulator
- Model trimmer
- Plaster of Paris
- Elastic band
- Plaster bowl, spatula and knife
- Sticky wax
- Modelling clay

Work safety

Care should be taken when using the model trimmer to ensure that your fingers or any other part of your body or clothing does not come into contact with the wheel. Eye protection should be worn at all times when using the model trimmer.

Basic procedure

1. Set the incisal pin to its 0° position and lock the condyles into the hinging position. Position the mounting plates or nuts as required.

2. Check that the rims fit accurately on to each model independently and when arranged together. Double check that the heels of the models are not interfering.

3. Ensure the registration rims are securely attached to each other and the models.

4. The sides of the models are tapered (approximately 20°) along the front, sides, back and corners on the model trimmer, or the bases grooved to allow the models to be repositioned if removed (split-cast mounting technique).

Continued over

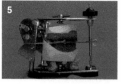
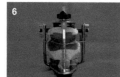
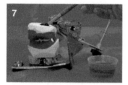
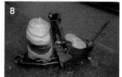
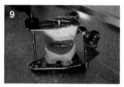
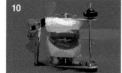
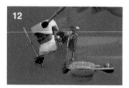
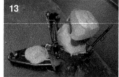
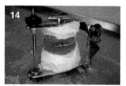
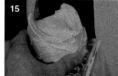
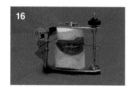

5. Use three mounds of modelling clay on the lower arm of the articulator to support the models in position within the articulator to conform to the Bonwill triangle.

6. Adjust the position such that the occlusal plane (contacting surfaces of the rims) and centre line of the lower rim just contact the incisal indicator pin, and the occlusal plane corresponds to an elastic band placed around the articulator and into the notches provided.

7. Coat the top and tapered sides of the maxillary model with two layers of plaster-separating solution.

8. With the articulator open, mix plaster and place on the upper model trying to create a tall mound – this will avoid plaster spilling over the sides of the model. Place plaster carefully around the mounting plate or nut. Close the articulator gently and ensure that the incisal pin is contacting the table.

9. Use a plaster knife to fill any remaining gaps between the articulator and model. The plaster will be neatened on the model trimmer later.

10. Allow to set for at least 10 minutes.

11. Turn the articulator upside down and remove the modelling clay.

12. Apply two layers of plaster-separating solution to the base of the mandibular model.

13. Mix plaster and place on the lower articulating plate and base of the mandibular model. Close the articulator gently and ensure that the incisal pin is contacting the table.

14. Use a plaster knife to fill any remaining gaps between the articulator and model.

15. When set the mounting plaster and models can be removed from the articulator and trimmed smooth on the model trimmer.

16. Replace the models back onto the articulator, and check that, with the registration rims in place, the incisal pin is touching the table.

Hints and tips

It is not always possible to contact the lower rim with the incisal indicator pin; therefore, the upper centre line/occlusal plane is used and a slight error in position accepted.

Secondary impression taking > Secondary impression casting > Registration rims production

1.20 Articulating models using a facebow

Facebows establish the relationship between the teeth and the condyles, or in edentulous cases, between the maxilla/mandible and the condyles.

Different designs of facebows record the relationship between either the mandible or the maxilla and the condyles. Facebows can be used either on the maxilla or on the mandible.

The facebow is used to position the respective model on the articulator so that the relationship between the patient's teeth (or edentulous ridges) and their condyle heads can be replicated on the articulator.

You will need:

- Models
- Transfer jig (from the clinician) – affixed to occlusal registration
- Denar articulator
- Model trimmer
- Plaster of Paris
- Elastic band
- Plaster bowl, spatula and knife
- Sticky wax

Work safety

Care should be taken when using the model trimmer to ensure that your fingers or any other part of your body or clothing does not come into contact with the wheel. Eye protection should be worn at all times when using the model trimmer.

Basic procedure

1. The bases of the models are tapered (split-cast mounting technique) as for the average-value mounting technique.

2. The upper or lower model (depending on whether a mandibular or maxillary facebow is used) is then attached to the bitefork of the facebow (in dentate patients the impression of the teeth is attached to the bitefork, and in edentulous patients the occlusal rim is attached to the fork).

3. The facebow is then adjusted to correspond to the articulator so as to be in the same relationship to the articulator as it was when positioned to the patient's skull, in relation to the condyle heads.

4. The mandibular facebow is supplied with a stand, the facebow is attached to the stand by a universal joint, via this joint the facebow can be adjusted until the correct relationship is achieved, that is, so that the pencil pointers are pointing to the centre of the condylar elements of the articulator (Condylator articulator).

5. Maxillary facebows have a pad or cup arrangement, which is positioned to correspond to the patient's condyle heads. This type of facebow does not have a stand but a height adjustment leg.

6. In use, an orbital pointer is adjusted to correspond to the lower orbit of one of the patient's eyes; when the pads or cups of the facebow have been positioned onto the condyle head elements of the articulator, the height is achieved by adjusting the height leg until the orbit pointer touches the orbital indicator plate on the upper arm of the articulator (Dentatus).

7. Some maxillary facebows (Denar) should be more accurately described as earbows as the condyle head pointers are designed to fit into the patient's ears.

8. These earbows usually incorporate a transfer jig, which, after the earbow has been positioned and secured, can be detached from the earbow, carrying the bitefork.

9. The transfer jig is then placed into a special locating hole in the incisal guidance element of the articulator, the bitefork being in

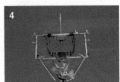
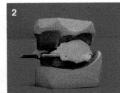
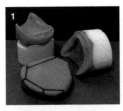
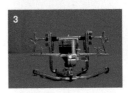
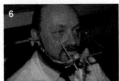
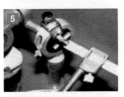
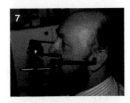
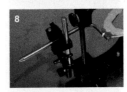
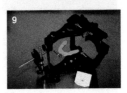

Continued over

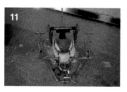
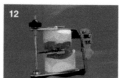

the same relationship to the condyle heads of the articulator as it was to the patient's condyle heads.

10. To ensure that no unwanted movement occurs, it is essential that irrespective of the type of transfer bow used, the clinician ensures that all locking devices are secure before transfer to the laboratory.

11. Having adjusted and correctly positioned the facebow to the articulator, the upper or lower models can be secured to the bitefork (via the occlusal block or bite registration) with sticky wax and attached to the articulator with plaster of Paris.

12. Once set, the facebow can be removed, the opposing model positioned using the occlusal record provided (plaster keys or silicone wafer), attached with sticky wax and plastered to the articulator.

Extended information

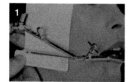
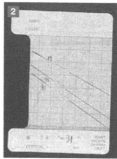
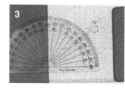

Recording the condylar angle

Condylar angle recordings are taken (protrusive or right and left lateral) with wax or silicone wafers in the case of the Dentatus and Denar, or using pencil tracing or condylar movements as with the Condylator mandibular facebow). These readings can be calculated/measured and put into the condylar elements of the articulator.

Condylar angle recording using pencil tracings with a mandibular facebow:

1. After the registration procedures have been completed and the facebow positioned correctly, a graph card is positioned around the patient's ear parallel to the horizontal arm of the facebow.

2. The pencil marker is released gently onto the graph card and the patient instructed to make a protrusive movement of the mandible. The clinician should ensure the card is kept still and parallel to the horizontal arm of the facebow during this procedure.

3. Three tracings are carried out per side. The tracings are measured using a protractor after first drawing tangents to the curves, with the mean of the three tracings being used to determine the left and right condylar angles. The condylar head elements of the articulator can then be adjusted to these angles.

Condylar angle recording using silicone templates or wafers with maxillary facebows:

Continued over

1. After the registration procedures have been completed, but before the blocks are sealed together, notches are cut in both the upper and lower registration blocks and the upper registration block is placed in the mouth. A layer of silicone registration paste is placed on the lower block.

2. With the lower block in the mouth, the patient is asked to move the jaw to the right lateral position and close the registration blocks together. The blocks are removed and separated from the silicone template, and the process is repeated to record the left lateral occlusion. It is possible to take just one protrusive record to give the forward positions of both condyles at the same time instead of the left and right lateral ones.

3. To set the condylar angle, loosen the articulator condylar screw and replace the retrusive, or protrusive, template between the record blocks.

4. Move the upper arm of the articulator and the adjustable condylar path element of the articulator until the template is accurately seated between the registration blocks. Lock the condylar element on the side opposite to that to which the mandible has moved (non-working side).

5. Repeat the procedure with the other lateral template. If the protrusive template has been used, the procedure is the same except that both condylar elements are adjusted and fixed at the same time.

6. It should be noted that wafer techniques are susceptible to inter-operator variability.

Hints and tips

When closing the articulator onto the plaster on the upper model, support the bitefork and ensure that the incisal pin is touching the mounting jig. Hold for a moment until the plaster relaxes.

Devices can be purchased to aid the support of the bitefork when in position as the weight of the model may cause the bitefork to move.

Chapter 2 | COMPLETE PROSTHETICS

2.1 Introduction to complete prosthetics

Complete prosthetics refers to the provision of complete or full dentures. The procedure for providing dentures consists of five key stages:

(1) **Primary impression** > *Manufacture of customised tray*

(2) **Secondary impression** > *Manufacture of registration rims*

(3) **Occlusal registration** > *Set-up of teeth*

(4) **Try-in** > *Processing of denture*

(5) **Fitting**

(Note: The clinical stages are indicated in **bold**, and those conducted in the dental laboratory in *italics*.)

Primary impressions are discussed in Chapter 1; here, we begin with the manufacture of a customised tray.

Overview of custom impression trays

Custom impression trays are used to overcome the inaccuracies associated with primary impressions. They are custom-made to fit the denture-bearing area on the primary model. Their design and accurate fit allows for better control of impression materials that are fluid and must be guided into place. Similarly to stock trays, they are used to support and transport the impression material to the mouth and once set, to the laboratory. The design of the tray will depend on the amount of undercut present and the type of impression material being used.

A well-designed impression tray should

- support the impression material in contact with the oral tissues;

- allow pressure to be applied by the clinician on selected areas of the denture-bearing area;

- retain its shape throughout the impression procedure and during model production.

In edentulous cases, the majority of denture-bearing areas are free from large undercuts and impressions may be taken in close-fitting trays using impression materials which are rigid (non-elastic) when set, that is, zinc oxide and eugenol paste.

When undercuts are present, spacing is required. The amount depends on the amount of undercut to be recorded, the elastic limit and the tear strength of

Basics of Dental Technology: A Step By Step Approach, Second Edition.
Tony Johnson, David G. Patrick, Christopher W. Stokes, David G. Wildgoose and Duncan J. Wood.
© 2016 John Wiley & Sons, Ltd. Published 2016 by John Wiley & Sons, Ltd.
Companion Website: www.wiley.com/go/johnson/basicsdentaltechnology

the chosen impression material. A weak material such as alginate requires more spacing than a tough material such as silicone.

Spacing is also required for stiff (high viscosity) impression materials because unless there is some spacing between the tray and the tissues it is difficult to seat the tray without using considerable force. There are few indications in complete denture prosthetics for the use of such high viscosity materials for working impressions.

The information you should find on the prescription card and impression is as follows:

- Type of tray required, that is, close-fitting/spaced

- Type of handle required

- The outline (peripheral extension) required for the custom-made tray. This is drawn on the primary impression by the clinician with an indelible pencil for alginate or a permanent marker pen for silicone. This should transfer to the model on casting.

Materials for tray construction

Light-curing composite blanks are the most common and easy to use materials for tray construction. They are supplied in a uniform thickness and are dimensionally stable on curing and in storage. They are more expensive than self-curing acrylic. However, although self-curing acrylic resin is cheap, it has limited working time and easily distorts during curing.

Shellac is a form of wax which softens on heating. It is easy to adjust but is brittle, may distort at relatively low temperatures and is less easy to use.

Heat-cured acrylic resin is accurate and stable during use; however, it is very expensive in terms of the time taken to manufacture.

Primary impression casting ⟩ Customised tray construction ⟩ Secondary impression casting

2.2 Construction of a close-fitting custom impression tray

Introduction

To take an accurate impression of the patient's oral tissues, a custom-made tray is constructed to support the impression material (Figure 2.2.1).

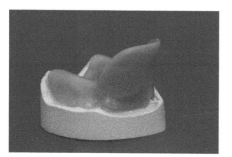

Figure 2.2.1

Work safety

The main risks associated with custom tray construction relate to the handling of the light-curing composite blanks. These materials can cause skin irritation and surgical gloves should be worn when handling these materials. Wash hands thoroughly after use.

You will need:

- A primary model
- A prescription card from the clinician
- Bunsen burner
- Wax carver/knife
- Tungsten carbide burs
- Sandpaper and mandrel

- Modelling wax
- Plaster-separating solution
- Light-curing tray material
- Light-curing box
- Scissors
- Yellow soft paraffin BP (Vaseline)
- Light-curing varnish (optional)

Basic procedure

1. If the peripheral outline has not been transferred from the impression to the model, draw the outline of the tray on the model at the deepest part of the sulcus, keeping clear of the muscle attachments.

2. Fill any undercuts with molten denture wax.

3. Coat the model with a layer of plaster-separating solution and allow to dry.

4. Adapt a sheet of light-curing tray material closely to the model; avoid thinning the material.

5. Trim to the marked outline of the tray. Keep the excess for making the handle. Although light-cured tray materials have a long working time, they will partially harden under strong light, so ensure they are stored in a sealed dark box.

6. Place the tray in a light box and cure following the manufacturer's instructions. Remove the tray from the model after curing and repeat on the underside ensuring full curing of the material (the light only penetrates to a depth of 1–2 mm).

7. Trim the periphery of the tray using an acrylic trimming bur to produce a rounded profile. Care should be taken to ensure that no sharp edges are left on the tray (if it feels sharp against your hand it will feel very sharp against the oral tissues).

8. After trimming, fit the tray base back onto the model and check that the peripheral extension matches the pencil line drawn on the model.

9. Form the tray handle from the surplus material. The handle should extend to the premolar regions and occupy the space of the natural teeth (see Extended information for handle designs).

10. Ensure the handle and base are well blended and then cure the tray for a second time to fix the handle.

11. Remove the tray from the model and trim the handle to shape.

12. Sandpaper may be used to smooth the surface if required.

13. Wash the tray using soapy water and steam clean the model to remove any blocking out wax.

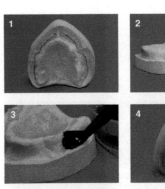
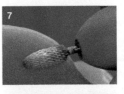
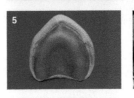
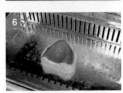
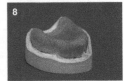
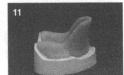
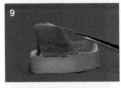
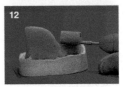

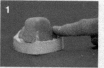
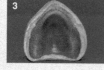

Custom trays made from light-cured materials can look unfinished even after extensive sandpapering. To improve the finished appearance:

1. Rub Vaseline into the surface of the finished tray until completely covered.

2. Light cure the tray in the light box.

3. Remove any excess Vaseline with boiling water. The surface finish will now be much improved.

Alternatively, some manufacturers supply a finishing varnish to give the light-cured material a smooth, glossy finish. This is applied and light cured after the tray is completed.

To improve the grip on the handle of the tray during use (the handle can become slippery and hard to grip when wet) a hot wax knife blade can be drawn across the handles to create a ridged groove.

Extended information

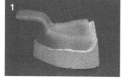
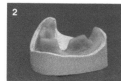

Handle design

Different handle types may be requested to suit the preference of the clinician.

- An intra-oral handle (as described above).

- An extra-oral stepped handle for an edentulous mouth.

- Finger stop handles are sometimes preferred for close-fitting trays.

2.3 Construction of a tray with spacer for edentulous cases

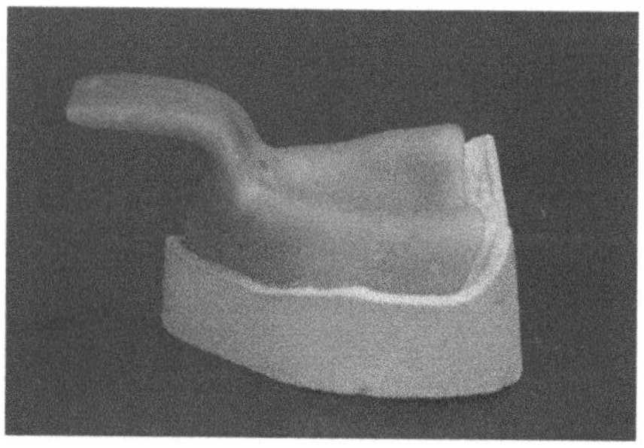

Introduction

Figure 2.3.1

Spaced trays (Figure 2.3.1) are used with alginate and elastomeric impression materials when undercuts are to be recorded. The material must be adequately thick to allow elastic deformation on removal from an undercut and avoid permanent distortion. Alginate, particularly, has low tear strength and must be used in thick sections.

Basic procedure

1. Adapt softened modelling wax onto the model and trim them 1–2 mm short of the required peripheral depth. This ensures that the sulcus is recorded entirely by the impression material. For alginate impression material place two layers of wax, and for silicones place one layer (and two where a deep undercut is located).

2. The exposed surfaces of the model should be coated in plaster-separating solution prior to applying the tray material.

3. Apply a light-curing acrylic blank over the wax spacers and trim with a knife to the edge of the wax.

4. Light cure in a light box.

5. An extra-oral stepped handle is provided on this type of tray.

6. The tray should be finished (including the handle) and trimmed to shape as described for close-fitting custom trays.

7. To provide mechanical retention, trays for alginate impressions need to have perforations. The tray produced should have 2 mm diameter holes drilled into it at 10-mm intervals. Do not place holes within 2 mm of the periphery of the tray in case minor adjustments to the edge of the tray are needed.

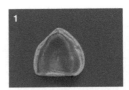
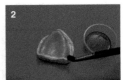
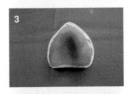
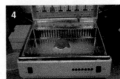
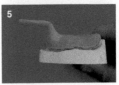
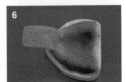
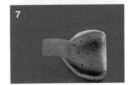
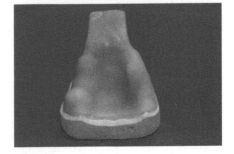

2.4 Construction of a tray for dentate or partially dentate cases

Primary impression casting → Customised tray construction → Secondary impression casting

Introduction

Spaced trays are used with alginate and elastomeric impression materials when undercuts are to be recorded (Figure 2.4.1). The material must be adequately thick to allow elastic deformation on removal from an undercut and avoid permanent distortion. Alginate, particularly, has low tear strength and must be used in thick sections.

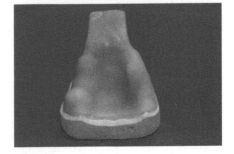

Figure 2.4.1

You will need:

- A primary model
- A prescription card from the clinician
- Bunsen burner
- Wax carver/knife
- Tungsten carbide burs
- Sandpaper and mandrel
- 2-mm rosehead bur

- Modelling wax
- Plaster-separating solution
- Light-curing tray material
- Light-curing box
- Scissors
- Yellow soft paraffin BP (Vaseline)
- Light-curing varnish (optional)

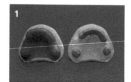
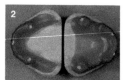
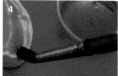
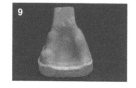

Basic procedure

1. Adapt softened modelling wax sheets onto the model to cover the teeth. Trim to 3 mm past the gingival margin.

2. Adapt a second sheet over the entire model and trim 1–2 mm short of the required peripheral depth. This ensures that the sulcus is recorded entirely by the impression material. See Table 2.4.1 for wax spacer thicknesses.

3. If the clinician has requested occlusal or tooth stops, see Extended information below.

4. The exposed edges of the model should be coated in plaster-separating solution prior to applying the tray material.

5. The tray construction is identical to that described in Section 2.3 for an edentulous tray with spacer.

6. A light-curing acrylic blank is applied over the wax spacers and trimmed with a knife to the edge of the wax and light cured.

7. An extra-oral handle is provided on this type of tray and is stepped if the anterior section is edentulous.

8. The tray should be finished (including the handle) and trimmed to shape as described for spaced trays.

9. To provide mechanical retention, trays for alginate impressions need to have perforations. The tray produced should have 2-mm diameter holes drilled into it at 10-mm intervals. Do not place holes within 2 mm of the periphery of the tray in case minor adjustments to the edge of the tray are needed. If silicone impression materials are to be used, no perforations are necessary.

Table 2.4.1 Space requirement for impression materials

Impression material	Space required
Zinc oxide and eugenol paste	No spacer wax (0.5–1 mm)
Silicone (medium bodied)	1.5–3 mm (one layer of wax)
Alginate	3 mm (two layers of wax)
Silicone (heavy bodied)	3–4.5 mm (three layers of wax)
Impression plaster	4.5 mm (three layers of wax)

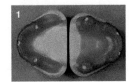

2.5 Construction of a windowed close-fitting tray

Introduction

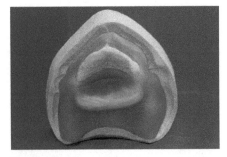

There are occasions when a close-fitting special tray would be desirable, but is contraindicated due to the presence of a section of flabby ridge. The problem is overcome by the use of a close-fitting tray with a window cut in the tray around the fibrous ridge area (Figure 2.5.1). This design enables a close-fitting impression to be taken of the firm areas of the mouth, whilst impression plaster can be used to record the fibrous part.

Figure 2.5.1

You will need:

- A primary model
- A prescription card from the clinician
- Bunsen burner
- Wax carver/knife
- Tungsten carbide burs
- Sandpaper and mandrel
- Modelling wax
- Plaster-separating solution
- Light-curing tray material
- Light-curing box
- Scissors
- Yellow soft paraffin BP (Vaseline)
- Light-curing varnish (optional)

Work safety

The main risks associated with custom tray construction relate to the handling of the light-curing composite blanks or self-curing acrylic resin. These materials can cause skin irritation and surgical gloves should be worn when handling these materials. Wash hands thoroughly after use.

Basic procedure

1. The flabby ridge section should have been indicated by the clinician on the primary impression. Mark this on the model.

2. Construct the tray base as for the close-fitting tray (see Section 2.2).

3. Trim the material around the flabby ridge as indicated using a knife prior to light curing.

4. The tray handle is placed across the palate in the premolar region (the fibrous areas are usually in the anterior region). The tray is cured again and finished as for the close-fitting tray.

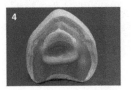

Secondary impression casting ▶ Registration rims production ▶ Articulating models

2.6 Construction of occlusal registration rims

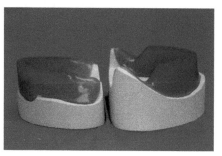

Figure 2.6.1

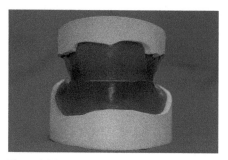

Figure 2.6.2

Introduction

Occlusal registration rims (also known as wax rims, or bite blocks (Figures 2.6.1 and 2.6.2) are used by the clinician to record all the information from the patient that is required to construct the trial dentures.

Six pieces of information are recorded using the registration rims:

(1) Occlusal plane: the plane at which the teeth meet

(2) Lip support: the labial surface of the denture teeth

(3) Centre line: midline of the face that will be used to position the teeth

(4) High 'smile line': the extent of the teeth and mucosa shown during a smile

(5) Vertical dimension: the height required for the dentures

(6) Centric relation: jaw relationship required for the dentures.

For further details see the Extended information box. The dimensions used in the following instructions are based on average values found in clinical situations.

Work safety

The main risks associated with custom tray construction relate to the handling of the light-curing composite blanks. These materials can cause skin irritation and surgical gloves should be worn when handling these materials. Wash hands thoroughly after use.

You will need:

- Working models
- A prescription card
- Bunsen burner
- Light-curing composite blanks
- Denture wax
- Preformed wax rim (optional)
- An occlusal rim inclinator

- Wax carver/knife
- Plaster-separating solution
- Light-curing box
- Ruler
- Cotton wool, lemon oil (or other suitable wax solvent) and liquid soap

Basic procedure

1. Fill the undercuts on the models with molten denture wax and coat the model with two layers of plaster-separating solution. Leave to dry.

2. Adapt a light-curing composite sheet to the upper model. Trim the excess to reveal the land area of the model. The base should extend to fill the entire sulcus, or to the extension indicated by the clinician.

3. The lower is constructed in the same way, ensuring that the material is bulky enough to resist fracture.

4. Cure the material in the light-curing box (cure both sides to ensure complete curing).

5. Remove the cured baseplates from the model. Trim any excess material or rough edges using a tungsten carbide bur, then sandpaper them smooth.

6. To aid retention of the wax rim, sticky wax may be added to the crest of the base (pass the Bunsen burner over the sticky wax to melt it just prior to placing the wax rim) or the surface may be roughened using a bur.

7. Soften a preformed wax rim in warm water until pliable. Dry the wax and position over the baseplate so that the labial surface replicates the lost teeth (over the ridge in the mandible and slightly forward of the ridge in the maxilla). (A wax rim can be made by tightly rolling three-quarters of a sheet of softened modelling wax if you do not have preformed rims – see Hints and tips).

8. Squeeze the wax rim onto the base between the fingers and thumb to adapt it closely.

9. Using a hot wax knife, seal the wax rim to the base with denture wax.

10. Placing a pencil mark on the outside of the models level with the lowest point of the sulcus, next to the central fraenum.

11. On the maxillary model use the pencil mark as a reference point and measure 22 mm and record using a wax knife to establish the anterior level of the rim.

12. Repeat for the mandibular rim, but using 18 mm as the rim height.

13. Now adjust the occlusal plane: heat the rim inclinator in a Bunsen burner. The right-angled edge of the plate is then placed across the hamular notches.

14. The hot plate is then rotated towards the wax rim, keeping the inclinator plate in contact with the hamular notches at all times.

Continued over

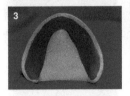
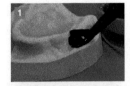
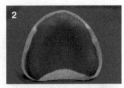
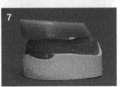
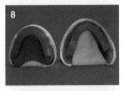
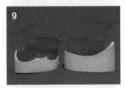
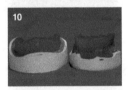
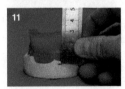
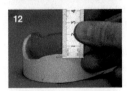
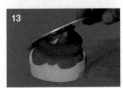
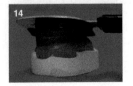

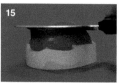
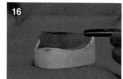
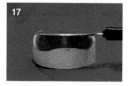
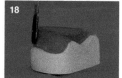
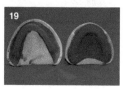
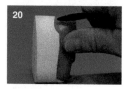
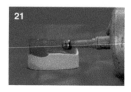
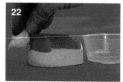
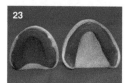

15. Continue until the excess wax has been removed to the desired height determined previously.

16. For the mandibular rim adjust the height to 18 mm anteriorly and level with a point two-thirds the way up the retromolar pads. Draw a line between these two points with a wax knife.

17. Melt away the excess using a knife or the inclinator as a hot plate.

18. Shape and smooth the sides of both rims using a wax knife.

19. The rim width should be between 5 and 7 mm anteriorly and between 7 and 8 mm posteriorly.

20. Contour the outer surfaces to blend the wax into the baseplate.

21. Finish the wax surface by passing the flame of the Bunsen burner quickly across the wax to just melt the surface and make it smooth.

22. Alternatively, a wax solvent, such as lemon oil, can be applied to smooth the surface.

23. Finish the registration rims by scoring the tops of the rims across a piece of sandpaper on a flat surface. Polish the finished rims with cotton wool and soapy water if desired.

Hints and tips

Baseplates are often produced using wax with a wire strengthener or using shellac rather than the light-cured composite. Although cheaper than light-curing bases these materials distort in the mouth and can lead to an incorrect registration. A re-try as a result of distortion requires an extra clinical visit and is expensive in terms of time.

Prior to carving, smoothing or polishing the wax, cool the rims in cold water for a few minutes to harden the wax.

Preformed rims may be made in the laboratory either by pouring molten scrap wax into a mould or they may be bought from a dental supplier.

When making a rim from a sheet of wax, soften this over a Bunsen flame without melting the surface. Fold 1 cm of the sheet over and gently squeeze out any air. Repeat until you reach the end of the sheet. Use immediately whilst still soft.

Extended information

Wax registration rims are often poorly constructed. The technique described above is time efficient and produces blocks that are anatomically well designed. If the rims are made to these 'average' dimensions and anatomical angles, the registration process will be easier, quicker and more accurately carried out.

Occlusal rim width is a feature often ignored during construction. Wide rims restrict the tongue space and encroach into the cheeks and lips, distorting the denture-bearing area. This can lead to movement of the rims during registration, resulting in inaccurate registration of the occlusion. In general, rims should be slightly wider than the teeth they will eventually carry.

The information recorded on the rims by the clinician is used to construct the trial dentures. Below is a brief description of what is recorded, how it is recorded and why.

Lip support

The labial lip support is determined by looking at the lip support and facial contour as well as checking for encroachment on the tongue. Wax is added or removed from the rim until correct.

Continued over

This primarily determines the position of the teeth labially. During positioning of the teeth, the labial surface of the rim will be followed. Having the teeth in the correct position bucco-lingually is important to aid retention and stability as the soft tissues can hold the denture in place and the forces transmitted through the teeth are directed centrally over the alveolar ridge.

Occlusal plane

Using the upper lip as an initial guide the level of the incisal edges of the upper central incisor teeth are scribed on to the rim. This position is then used as the anterior reference point of the occlusal plane. Using a Fox's guide plane as an aid, the rim is adjusted so that the occlusal plane is parallel to the ala-tragus line (Camper's line).

The occlusal plane is the plane to which the teeth are placed to meet or occlude. Reasonable accuracy is required to allow enough room for both upper and lower teeth to be positioned. The relationship to the condyle must be correct for a balanced occlusion and good aesthetics.

Vertical dimension

The vertical dimension is the height of the rims when in contact. It is determined by establishing an adequate freeway space (difference between occlusal face height and rest face height). An over-provision of freeway space would allow the patient to over-close. This causes poor aesthetics and possibly temporomandibular joint (TMJ) problems. If not excessively worn, the old set of dentures is a good indicator.

The vertical dimension establishes the tooth position on the trial dentures. It is important that the patient has space between the teeth when relaxing and that they do not over-close on biting. Correct vertical dimension also gives support to facial tissues, preventing creasing at the corner of the mouth.

In a case with a high smile line, this is marked to indicate where the upper lip will be when the patient is smiling, to allow for this in the placement of the teeth and to avoid leaving too much visible gum.

Centre line

This is marked on the rims in line with the centre of the patient's face, allowing the teeth to be positioned centrally for symmetry.

Centric relation

The patient is asked to touch their soft palate with the tip of their tongue and close their teeth together to the retruded contact position (RCP). This ensures the condyle is in the correct position in the TMJs. The rims are sealed together in this position.

This records the relationship between the maxillae and mandible when the condyle is ideally positioned in the glenoid fossae. The denture teeth will then be set to create an intercuspal position (ICP) that coincides with the RCP.

The use of gothic arch tracing devices is recommended as being the most predictable and accurate method of recording centric relation.

2.7 Setting up denture teeth

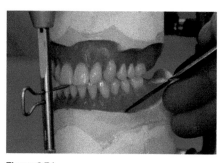

Figure 2.7.1

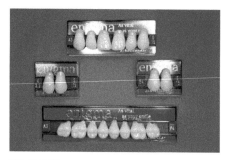

Figure 2.7.2

Introduction

The aim is to place the denture teeth on the registration rims to conform to the recordings made by the clinician in a position that is both functional and aesthetically pleasing (Figure 2.7.1).

The shape, size and shade of the teeth are chosen by the clinician to harmonise with the patient's stature, sex, size, age and complexion (Figure 2.7.2). (See Extended information for more details.)

The teeth are arranged such that a balanced occlusion is established. A balanced occlusion is an occlusal scheme designed to make the denture stable during function. Each tooth should contact the opposing tooth in the ICP. This means that the teeth meet at the occlusal plane.

In lateral movements of the mandible, the teeth should contact on the working side and there should also be contact between the palatal cusps of the upper and buccal cusps of the lower teeth on the balancing side. This ensures that the denture will not tip during function. Similarly, when protruding the mandible, there should be contact between the anterior teeth and some posterior teeth on both sides.

Work safety

Care should be taken when working with a Bunsen burner and hot wax. When grinding the acrylic teeth use dust extraction and wear eye protection.

You will need:

- Prescription (which may include photographs and impressions of the patient's old dentures or diagrams)
- Denture teeth, matching the prescription
- Registration rims
- Upper and lower models mounted on an articulator
- Wax carver/knife

- Glass slab
- Denture wax
- Bunsen burner
- Pencil
- Tungsten burs (large and small)
- Articulating paper
- Cotton wool and lemon oil (or other suitable wax solvent) optional

Basic procedure

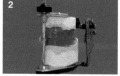

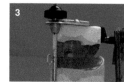

1. Place the models on the articulator and ensure that the centric lock is engaged, and that the incisal pin is in contact with the incisal table. This should remain so through all steps of the following procedure.

2. Transcribe the centre line from the upper to the lower rim.

3. Using a hot wax knife remove a section of wax from the wax rim to make room for an upper central incisor.

Continued over

4. Soften the wax within the cut region and position the central incisor flush with the labial contour of the wax block, just touching the occlusal plane (the junction of the upper and lower blocks).

5. A glass slab may be used to indicate the occlusal plane, and so aid the positioning of the teeth.

6. If room for the tooth is limited, the baseplate can be reduced in thickness using a tungsten bur. If this is not sufficient the neck of the tooth can also be removed.

7. The long axis of the tooth should be vertical when viewed labially and proclined when viewed from the distal aspect.

8. Repeat the procedure for the adjacent lateral incisor. It should be rotated such that the long axis of the tooth is no longer vertical but raised by 1 mm off of the occlusal plane. However, for older patients the lateral incisor should be level with the occlusal plane (see Figures 7a and 7b).

9. Position the adjacent canine such that it shows only its mesial aspect when viewed from the front. The long axis of the tooth should be vertical when viewed from the labial aspect. The neck of the canine should be prominent.

10. The teeth should form a smooth arch when viewed occlusally.

11. Repeat steps 2–10 to complete the opposite side.

Objectives of setting the posterior teeth

Position the upper posterior teeth slightly buccal to the alveolar ridge, conforming to the compensating curve. The diagrams 11b, 11c and 11d show how this can be achieved by assessing the relationship between the occlusal plane and individual cusps on the teeth. The steepness of the curve depends on the condylar angle, cusp angle of the teeth and incisal guidance table. The average 30° condylar angles are usually used. Shallow cusped posterior teeth are generally preferred. Steep cusped teeth used with a 30° condylar angle requires inconveniently steep compensating curves if balanced articulation is to be achieved.

In a Class I occlusal relationship, the occlusal surfaces of the upper posterior teeth lie slightly buccal to the lower ridge allowing the palatal cusps to occlude with the lower fossae.

12. Remove the upper registration rim and mark the centre of the alveolar ridge using a pencil.

13. Extend this line to the edges of the model, so that when the baseplate is replaced, the line can still be seen. Using a cold wax knife, scribe this line onto the posterior of the wax rim.

14. Position the first premolar by cutting a small amount of wax from the rim. The premolar is positioned over the ridge such that its buccal and palatal cusps touch the occlusal plane.

15. Repeat the process for the second premolars, but only the palatal cusp should touch the occlusal plane with the buccal

Continued over

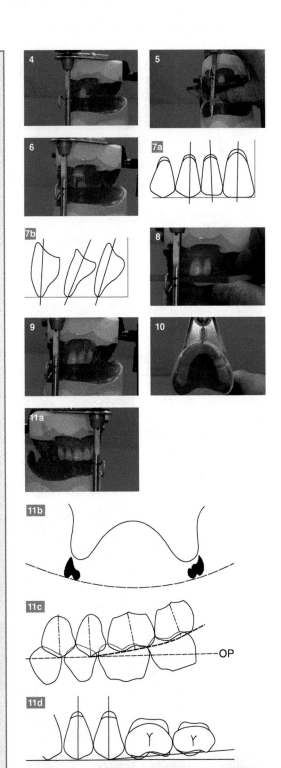
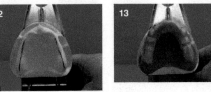
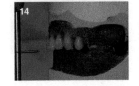

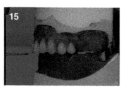
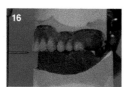

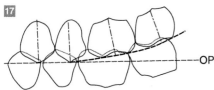
—OP

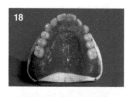
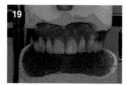

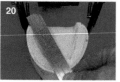
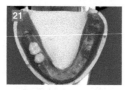

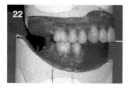
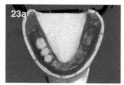

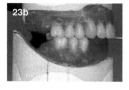
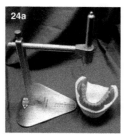

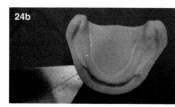

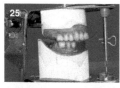
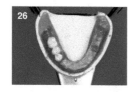

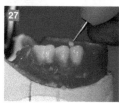
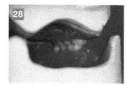

cusp about 1 mm away from the plane (which creates the compensating curve).

16. Position the first molar over the ridge such that the mesio-palatal cusp touches the occlusal plane and the buccal and distal cusps continue the compensating curve.

17. The second molars are optional, and should be placed where the buccal corridor allows them to be seen. The placing of the second molar often leads to instability of the denture. When placing a second molar, it should follow the compensating curves previously established by the second premolar and first molar.

18. Repeat steps 13–16 to complete the opposite side.

19. At this point, secure all the teeth into position by apply molten wax around the neck of the teeth.

20. The lower posterior teeth can now be set to the upper posterior teeth. As for the upper teeth, the aim is to position the teeth over the alveolar ridge. Remove the registration rim and mark the centre of the mandibular alveolar ridge using a pencil, and extend it to the model edges.

21. Replace the registration rim and scribe the line drawn above onto the wax rim. The central fossa of the lower teeth should align with this line (the centre of the alveolar ridge).

22. Start with the first molar. In a Class I skeletal relationship the mesio-palatal cusp of the upper first molar fits into the central fossa of the lower first molar (for other skeletal relationships, see Extended information). This dictates the position of the premolars. Never place molar teeth over sloping parts of the ridge, particularly the mandibular ridge. This causes the dentures to slide forwards when in function and subsequently to be unstable. This very often means leaving the second molars off the dentures.

23. Continue by placing the first and second premolars (23a and 23b).

24. In most cases, but particularly when it is essential to have the occlusal pressure exerted directly over the centre of the residual ridges, a laser may be used to ensure precise positioning of the posterior teeth (24a and 24b).

25. Use a wax knife to adjust the position of the lower teeth to ensure a firm occlusal contact. In difficult situations, teeth may be lightly adjusted at this stage to improve the occlusal contact. Place articulating paper (or silk) on the occlusal surface and gently close the articulator.

26. The contact points will be shown as ink marks.

27. Lightly reduce the contact to allow the other teeth to occlude (only grind the fossa, never the cusp tip).

28. The primary contact should be between the palatal cusp of the upper and the central fossa of the lower tooth. Contact also

Continued over

occurs between the buccal cusp of the lower and the fossa of the upper tooth.

29. Repeat steps 21–28 to complete the opposite side.

Objectives of setting the lower anterior teeth

Select the lower anterior teeth according to the space available between the premolars and to match the size of the upper incisors. For a Class I incisor relationship an overbite and overjet of 2 mm is recommended.

30. Position the lower central incisors with their necks on the alveolar ridge and the incisal edges proclined to create an ideal overbite and overjet of 2 mm (this may not always be possible but is not a problem as long as a balanced occlusion is created and the patient can function efficiently). Place the lower lateral incisors and canines to fill the available space.

31. In placing the lower anterior teeth, consideration should be given to the support they will give to the lip. However, care must be taken to avoid placing the lower anterior teeth such that the lower lip will be displaced and cause denture instability.

Final adjustments

32. On completing the positioning of the teeth and with occlusal contacts established, open the centric lock of the articulator.

33. Move the articulator into one lateral excursion and check that there is contact on the working side teeth. The canines may also need grinding to prevent canine guidance and allow group function.

34. Repeat step 33 for the opposite side.

35. Check the protrusive excursions to ensure contact between the anterior teeth.

36. The waxwork should be contoured to mimic the natural gingivae. Using a hot wax knife build up wax around the teeth to simulate the natural gingivae.

37. The wax is placed to simulate the canine and other eminences.

38. The wax around the teeth is carved back to reflect the age of the patient, that is, the older the patient the more the tooth should be revealed.

39. Ensure that no ledge is left around the teeth by rounding the gingival margin into the tooth.

40. The wax can then be smoothed with a Bunsen burner flame or by using a wax solvent.

41. The margins of teeth and wax should then be redefined.

42. The wax try-in can then be polished using damp cotton wool and soapy water.

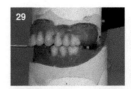
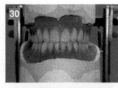
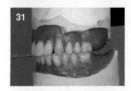
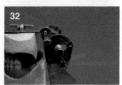
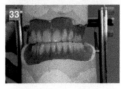
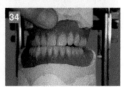
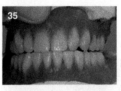
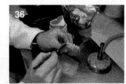
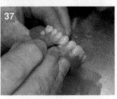
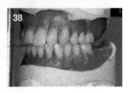
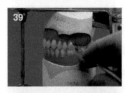
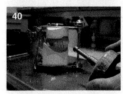
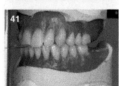
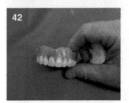

It is important to remember that where patients have Class II and III jaw relations the technician and clinician should not try to turn them into Class I denture relationships as this will lead to a loss of denture stability and often poor aesthetics.

For Class II relationships the lower posterior teeth are positioned half a unit distally to the Class I arrangement. This allows enough space for the anterior teeth to be positioned. The lower anterior teeth must still be positioned with their necks over the lower ridge. Any attempt to move them forward to 'correct' the incisor relationship will cause instability when the wearer attempts to incise food. The teeth can then be proclined to allow the patient to achieve edge-to-edge contact between the anterior teeth. In this Class II relationship, there is usually less room for the anterior teeth to be placed. It is better to place five correctly sized anterior teeth than to place six teeth that are too small.

For Class III relationships the lower posterior teeth should be positioned half a unit mesially to the class I arrangement. Class III jaw relations sometimes involve crossbites where a normal relationship is impossible. Here, only the lingual upper cusps need lie over the upper ridge. The lower anterior teeth should again be placed over the ridge and in contact with the upper incisors in centric occlusion. They may be proclined or straight, but retroclined arrangements should be avoided. In a Class III relationship there is usually too much room for the selected anterior teeth. In this case, it is better to place seven correctly sized teeth rather than selecting six teeth that are too big for the selected upper teeth.

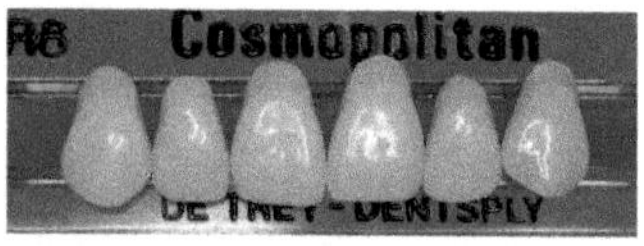

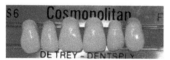

Figure 2.7.3

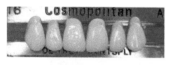

Figure 2.7.4

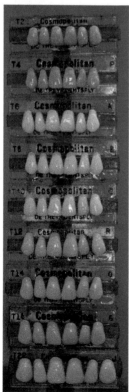

Figure 2.7.5

Figure 2.7.6

Aesthetics

Aesthetics is the art of arranging and positioning the teeth. It is possible, with the same mould and shade of tooth, to arrange them to show standard, masculine and feminine characteristics.

The arrangement and positioning of the teeth should be decided by the clinician and patient to complement the patient's sex, age, personality and skin tone. Communicating these decisions to the technician is difficult and therefore photographs, study models (of existing dentures) or diagrams should be used as an aid.

When the teeth are in their final position, the wax is made neat and corrected to match the set-up (the older the patient, the more tooth should be visible, etc.).

Tooth selection: choice of mould, size and shade of teeth

Three moulds of teeth are usually available: round, square or tapering, each in a range of sizes. The size of tooth chosen should harmonise with the patient's build.
Round (Figure 2.7.3**), square (Figure** 2.7.4**), tapered (Figure** 2.7.5**)**

Size comparison (Figure 2.7.6).

There are two methods of tooth shape selection. First, the shade is chosen to harmonise with the patient's complexion and age (the older the patient, usually the darker the teeth). Second, rounded teeth tend to have a more feminine or softer appearance whereas square teeth are often used to create a masculine appearance (Figure 2.7.7).

Occlusion

Two forms of posterior tooth relationship are popular for complete dentures: the natural (anatomical) occlusion and the lingualised occlusion.

The natural occlusion

Here, the upper teeth are placed in their natural position buccal to the crest of the ridge. Occlusion occurs between the palatal cusps of the upper and the central fossae of the lower as before, and the buccal cusps of the lower teeth and the central fossae of the upper.

The teeth also overlap each other as with natural teeth: the lower first premolar occluding with the upper canine and first premolar; the lower second premolar occluding with the upper premolars; and the lower first molar opposing the upper second premolar and first molar.

Final corrections for balance of the occlusal relationships in lateral and protrusive excursions are accomplished on each working side in turn using the BULL rule. The **B**uccal **U**pper cusps and the **L**ingual **L**ower cusps are adjusted to ensure that balancing side contacts between upper palatal and lower buccal cusps are maintained.

The lingualised occlusion

Here, the upper teeth are placed buccal to the upper ridge with occlusal contact between the palatal cusps of the upper teeth and the central fossae of the lower teeth. The first premolars differ in that the situation is reversed.

This form of tooth arrangement does not have any overlapping of the teeth as in the natural occlusion but has one upper tooth only occluding with its lower counterpart and not contacting any other lower teeth.

SQUARE   TAPERING   OVOID

Figure 2.7.7

2.8 Denture processing

Waxing up the denture → Flasking and packing → Finishing the denture

Introduction

The process involves the making of a two-part mould (flasking), the removal of the wax and replacement with acrylic (packing) and the removal from the mould and trimming of acrylic (finishing) (Figure 2.8.1).

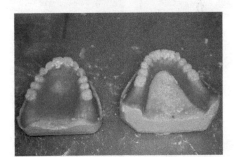

Figure 2.8.1

You will need:

- Plaster mixing bowl, spatula and knife
- Brush
- Copper-headed hammer
- Plaster saw
- Plaster of Paris and dental stone
- Denture-processing flasks and clamp
- Vaseline
- Plaster-separating solution
- Boiling water
- Heat-curing acrylic resin
- Water or dry-heat acrylic resin processing bath

Work safety

The mixing of acrylic resin products can be harmful to the operator. Gloves, facemask and protective eyewear should be worn. All acrylic resin products should be mixed in a fume cupboard or down draft extraction unit.

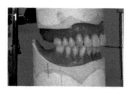
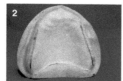
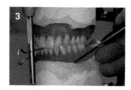
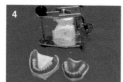
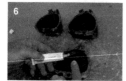
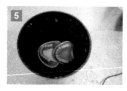
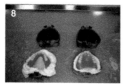
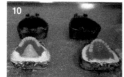
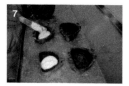
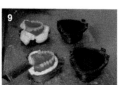
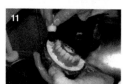
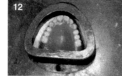
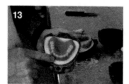
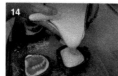
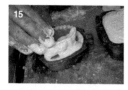
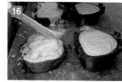
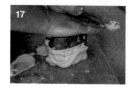
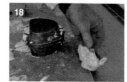

Basic procedure (flasking)

1.   With the dentures on the articulator, check that the tooth contacts and balanced occlusion are still satisfactory after the patient try-in.

2.   Check that the clinician has cut a post dam into the upper model. (If not, ensure that a post dam is not required.)

3.   With the wax dentures firmly seated and with the teeth in occlusion, seal the dentures to the model by running wax into the space between the wax dentures and the land area of the model.

4.   Remove the models from the articulating plaster by carefully tapping the sides of the articulating plaster. Do not use excessive force, or the model may get damaged.

5.   Place the models in water at room temperature for 5–10 minutes to remove air from the models.

6.   Coat the inside of two clean denture-processing flasks and inner sides of the end plates with a thin layer of Vaseline. Assemble the flasks to check that everything fits together without excessive force.

7.   Mix sufficient plaster of Paris to fill three-quarters of the two shallow halves of the denture flasks.

8.   Place the models into the plaster, positioning them so that the land area of the model is level with the edge of the flask.

9.   Trim the plaster so it fills the space between model and flask.

10. Bring the plaster up around the heels of the models and make sure no undercuts are present.

11. Smooth the plaster with a brush under running water as it reaches its initial set.

12. When the plaster has set completely, ensure that the two halves of the flask still meet properly.

13. Coat any exposed plaster or model with a thin layer of Vaseline. Care must be taken not to get Vaseline on the wax or teeth as this will result in a change in shape or tooth movement later in the process.

14. Mix 50:50 plaster and dental stone (Kaffir D) and fill the larger halves of the flasks.

15. Rub some of the remaining mix around the wax denture and the teeth with your fingers to prevent trapped air in the mould.

16. Tap the flask lightly on the bench to encourage the mix to flow into the detail of the denture. Place the remaining material over the denture to form a dome.

Continued over

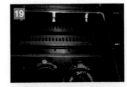
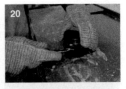
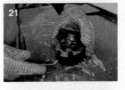
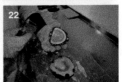
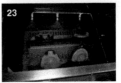
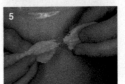

17. Turn the small half of the flask onto the larger half just before the initial set. Ensure the lugs engage and the two halves are pushed firmly together. Leave to set for at least 45 minutes. Avoid moving the flasks during setting as there is a danger of moving the flask plates. Whilst waiting, make sure that the boiling-out machine is on.

18. Once set, remove any excess plaster from the outside of the flasks.

19. Place the flasks in the heated boiling-out machine. Leave for approximately 5 minutes to allow the wax to soften.

20. Wearing protective gloves, remove and separate the two halves of the flasks and loosen gently all the way around the join using a plaster knife.

21. Once loose, lift the shallow half vertically to separate. Avoid twisting the two halves apart as you may damage the models.

22. Remove the baseplate and ensure that the teeth are secured in the plaster.

23. Replace the flask halves into the boiling-out machine to remove the remaining wax.

Basic procedure (packing)

1. Coat the plaster surfaces of the moulds with sodium alginate solution. This is best done when the plaster and stone are still warm. Remove any excess and allow to dry.

2. Avoid the material puddling around the teeth or other concave areas of the mould. Ensure that the teeth do not have any separator on them as this will prevent the acrylic resin bonding to the teeth and could lead to the teeth being detached from the denture base.

3. Mix the acrylic resin to the manufacturer's recommendations (this is typically a powder liquid ratio of 21 g:10 ml). Ensure that enough powder (polymer) is used to take up the excess liquid (monomer).

4. Mix the powder and liquid thoroughly to ensure there will be no dry powder particles (this is the cause of granularity). The mixing of the resin should take place in a vessel with a lid to prevent excess evaporation of the monomer, which can cause a dry, weak, mix.

5. The mix will go through various stages. Check the dough regularly to assess its progress. After the initial sandy consistency, the acrylic will become stringy when pulled.

Continued over

Hints and tips

During the wax removal from the flasks, care must be taken to ensure that no teeth become loose and are washed away down the sink or into the boiling-out machine. If teeth have loosened, they can be repositioned using a small spot of glue.

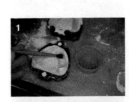
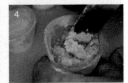
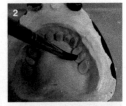
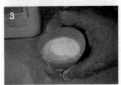
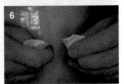
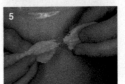

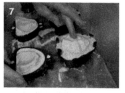
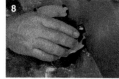

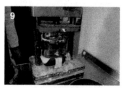
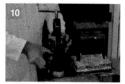

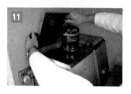
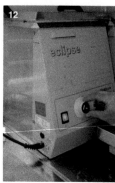

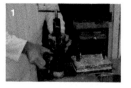
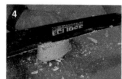

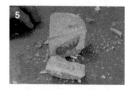
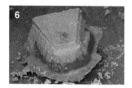

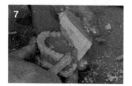
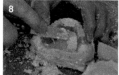
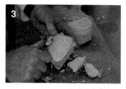
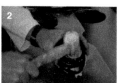

6. When the acrylic snaps cleanly when pulled, it is ready to be packed into the mould.

7. Place the resin into the larger half of the flask, where the teeth are, and press down firmly into the mould. Use an excess of material.

8. Place the smaller half of the flask, containing the model, on top and press down. Ensure the lugs are aligned.

9. Place the closed flasks in a bench press and slowly close one turn at a time until the two halves come together.

Note: There will always be a thin layer of acrylic resin between the two halves of the flask, called 'flash', no matter how much pressure is exerted. This will inevitably cause an increase in the vertical dimension and it is essential that care is taken to keep this to a minimum. A method to minimise the thickness of the flash is called a 'trial closure' and is described in the Extended information section below.

10. Place the flasks in a spring clamp and tighten.

11. Place the clamped flasks into a water or dry-heat curing bath (the water should be at room temperature before processing begins).

12. Set the delay timer to 5–7 hours at 70°C and the 'boiling' timer to 2–3 hours (at 100°C). This cure time (usually overnight) is long enough to cure the thickest denture. The long delay time will prevent any problems with gaseous porosity.

Basic procedure (finishing dentures)

1. Remove the flasks from the curing bath and clamps.

2. Tap the end plates on the flasks with a copper-headed hammer to remove the plaster mould from the flask.

3. Remove the white plaster from around the model by lightly tapping with a hammer. Remove any plaster adhering to the models with a plaster knife.

4. Starting with the upper denture, remove the 50:50 plaster from around the denture by cutting along the line of the teeth, taking care not to cut into the denture teeth.

5. When the cut is approximately 5 mm deep twist the saw blade sharply to break the side of the block away from the denture; repeat for the other side.

6. The plaster over the labial surface of the denture can be removed in the same way.

Continued over

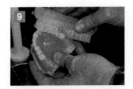

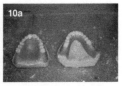

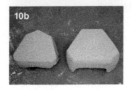

7. Gently prise the plaster from the palatal region using a plaster knife.

8. Repeat steps 4–7 for the lower denture.

9. Do not remove the dentures from the models at this stage. Clean the dentures and articulating surfaces of the models of plaster debris under the tap.

10. The dentures are now ready to be re-articulated.

Extended information

Trial closure

As previously mentioned trial closures can be performed to minimise the thickness of the flash. They are also carried out to allow staining of the labial surfaces of the dentures in certain techniques.

The technique involves separating the denture teeth or model from the acrylic resin when packing the denture. Placing a plastic or cellophane sheet over the teeth or model does this.

The resin is then packed into the two halves of the flasks as previously described and the two halves pressed together under pressure. The flasks can then be separated; the acrylic will be in the model or teeth half of the flask. The plastic or cellophane sheet can be removed and the flash removed with a sharp knife; any staining of the labial surfaces of the denture can be carried out if required.

The two halves of the flask are then placed together under the press and closed together and then clamped and cured as previously described.

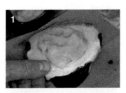

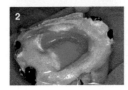

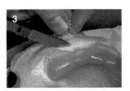

Porosity

There are two causes of porosity: polymerisation shrinkage, called contraction porosity, and volatilisation of the monomer, called gaseous porosity.

Contraction porosity

Contraction porosity occurs because the monomer contracts by around 20% of its volume during processing. By using the powder/liquid system, this contraction is minimised and should be around 5–8%. This is not translated into a high linear shrinkage, which, on the basis of the volumetric shrinkage, should be around 0.2–0.5%. At the curing temperature, the resin is able to flow into the spaces created by the curing contraction. The force of this flow is provided by the pressure exerted during the processing via a sprung clamp. Packing a slight excess of resin into the mould ensures that the resin is under pressure when the mould is closed and maintained during processing. It is therefore important that sufficient resin is packed into the mould for processing. This will cause any voids present in the mix to collapse, and should also help compensate for the curing contraction. The packing of the mould should only be carried out when the mix has reached the doughy

Continued over

stage; prior to this the high flow of the softer material causes a rapid loss of pressure.

Gaseous porosity
During polymerisation there is an exothermic reaction which can cause the temperature of the resin to rise above the boiling point of the monomer, which is 100.3°C. If this temperature is exceeded before the polymerisation process is finished, gaseous monomer is formed, creating porosities. The amount of heat depends on the volume of resin present, the proportion of monomer and the speed with which the external heat reaches the resin. Gaseous porosity can be avoided by allowing the temperature to be raised in a slow controlled way. The temperature is held at 70°C until the threat of an exothermic reaction has passed (5–7 hours) and then raised to 100°C for the final 2–3 hours of the curing cycle. Polymerisation of the acrylic resin should be carried out slowly to prevent gaseous porosity and under pressure to avoid contraction porosity.

Processing strains

The restriction imposed upon the dimensional change of the resin will give rise to internal strains. If these strains were allowed to relax, the result would be warpage, crazing and distortion of the denture base. Many of the strains generated during the curing contraction can be relieved by the flow of the resin above the glass transition temperature, but, some strains due to the thermal contraction will remain. The amount of internal strain can be reduced by using acrylic resin teeth instead of porcelain ones (preventing differential shrinkage on cooling) and by allowing the flasks to cool slowly. The relief of internal strain can produce tiny surface cracks called crazing, and can be seen as a hazy or foggy appearance of the surface of the resin. The crazing may be formed due to overheating during polishing, differential contraction around porcelain teeth or solvent attack. The introduction of cross-linked polymer chains into resins has reduced the potential for crazing.

Staining dentures

Stains can be added to the labial and buccal aspects of the dentures to provide a more realistic appearance. These come in the form of acrylic resin powders of various colours, which are carefully sprinkled onto the buccal and labial areas of the flasking plaster/stone and moistened with the accompanying liquid. Once the desired effects have been achieved the acrylic resin can be placed into the moulds as normal. The stains and the acrylic resin blend together during the curing cycle. (Staining is a relatively simple process but skill and practice are required to achieve predictable and accurate results.) Ethnic resins are available for use, usually coming in light, medium or dark shades. They are handled identically to standard resins and can also be stained if required.

Denture marking

Denture marking is a very good idea for dentures worn by patients who are likely to be hospitalised for regular periods or who live in retirement homes or who live in situations where their dentures could become mixed up with other patients' dentures.

There are a number of techniques available: The most modern is the embedded radio-frequency microchip. The other popular method is to print the patient's name onto onion paper or acetate sheet.

Continued over

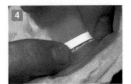

The microchip or onion paper or acetate sheet is then inserted into the denture after removing a small amount of the denture resin, the disto-buccal flange of the maxillary denture and the disto-lingual flange of the mandibular denture being the favoured sites. The device is then covered over with self-cured acrylic resin (4).

Injection packing of acrylic resin

This is a method of flasking and packing without any flash and therefore it does not increase the vertical dimension of the denture.

The wax try-ins are placed into the flasks as previously described in steps 1–23. The flasks are specially designed and have an entry hole at one end to allow the acrylic resin to be pressed into the mould. A connection between the wax denture and this hole is made using wax profiles before the investing procedure begins.

After investing and boiling out of the wax, any exposed plaster is coated with plaster-separating solution. Once the separating solution is dry the flasks can be secured together with the locking devices provided. The acrylic resin (either premixed or mixed conventionally and placed into a syringe) is then forced through the entry hole in the side of the flask under pressure until the mould is full. A pressure-maintaining device is then attached over the hole to ensure constant pressure during processing. The flasks can then be placed into the curing bath and cured as previously described.

2.9 Grinding and finishing the dentures

Waxing-up the denture   Flasking and packing   Finishing the denture

Introduction

The first stage in this process is to re-establish the occlusal contacts. This is necessary due to the increase in vertical dimension created during the flasking process and because teeth may move slightly in the plaster mould. See the following text regarding the occlusal scheme prior to commencing the procedure.

Once this is completed, the dentures are trimmed to remove any excess acrylic and polished to create an aesthetic and hygienic surface (Figure 2.9.1).

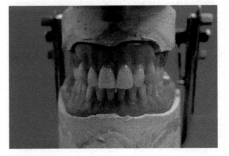

Figure 2.9.1

For natural occlusion: Care should be taken to preserve the cusps which provide the balancing side contacts (palatal upper and buccal of the lower). When removing premature contacts to achieve centric occlusion deepen the fossae rather than reducing the cusp height. Once centric occlusion is re-attained, the right and left lateral and protrusive excursions can be adjusted. Again, the buccal upper and lingual lower contacts are ground only (the BULL rule), in order to preserve balancing contacts.

For lingualised occlusion: The adjustment for centric occlusion is achieved by adjustment of the lower fossae and upper buccal cusps only as there is only one contact. When sliding into lateral and protrusive excursions the palatal upper cusps should be preserved. The lower buccal and lingual, and the upper buccal cusps may be ground.

You will need:

- Sodium citrate (plaster and stone solvent, if needed)
- Tungsten carbide burs, assorted stones, sandpaper mandrel and sandpaper strips
- Occlusal indicator cloth or paper
- Polishing machine, polishing mops and brushes
- Stippling bur
- Pumice and polishing compounds
- Denture pot or sealable plastic bag

Adjusting the occlusion should result in the teeth contacting in all excursions (as they did before processing) and the central articulator pin touching the incisal guidance table.

In any excursion, right, left, posterior and anterior, contacts should be maintained to achieve balance and stability.

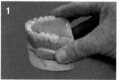

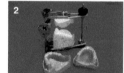

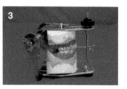

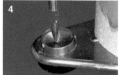

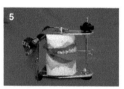

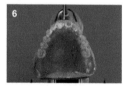

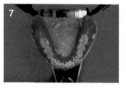

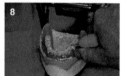

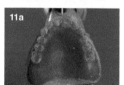

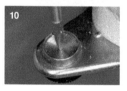

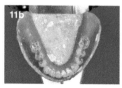

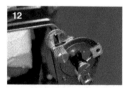

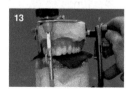

Basic procedure

1. Check that the models relocate accurately onto the articulating plaster mounts.

2. Place the articulating plaster back onto the articulator, and ensure that the condylar lock is engaged and that the incisal pin is set to 0.

3. Remount the models on the articulator using cyanoacrylate glue between the model and mounting plaster, or sticky wax along the joins. The fit between models and mounting plaster must be precise.

4. You may observe a change to the vertical dimension and occlusal contact (the articulator pin will not touch the table). This is a result of the flash between the two flask halves.

5. Place articulating paper (or silk) on the occlusal surfaces and close the articulator.

6. Open the articulator and observe the contacts recorded by the articulating paper.

7. The objective now is to reduce the increase in vertical dimension and simultaneously establish contacts on all posterior teeth.

8. Using a small bur, adjust the occlusal contacts minimally to reduce the vertical dimension. Note that reduction of 1 mm posteriorly is the equivalent of 3 mm anteriorly due to the hinging action of the jaw.

9. When grinding, avoid reducing the cusps that provide a balancing side contact in lateral excursions. These cusps are the palatal cusps of the upper, and the buccal cusps of the lower teeth.

10. Continue, repeatedly using articulating paper to check the contacts, until the vertical dimension is reduced (i.e. the pin touches the table).

11. Contact should occur between each opposing posterior tooth.

12. Open the centric locks on the articulator to allow the lateral and protrusive excursions to be checked.

13. With articulating paper on the occlusal surfaces, move the articulator into a right lateral excursion.

Continued over

14. The objective is to achieve contact on all the working side posterior teeth simultaneously; here, the lateral and canine are causing disclusion of the working side posterior teeth.

15. The contact is also causing disclusion of the balancing side teeth where contact between the palatal cusp of the upper and buccal cusp of the lower is required.

16. The articulating paper highlights the contacts. Reduce them to allow the posterior teeth to occlude in this excursion.

17. Continue identifying the contacts and reducing until the working side has contact on all teeth.

18. The incisal pin should contact the incisal table in the excursion.

19. Contacts should occur on the balancing side as well.

20. Repeat the procedure for left lateral excursion; here, the working side is shown.

21. Balancing side contacts between the upper palatal cusp and the lower buccal cusp should be achieved to ensure denture stability.

22. Check the protrusive excursion; the objective is to establish contacts on anterior and posterior teeth to avoid the denture tipping. Here, the anterior teeth are causing the posterior teeth to disclude.

23. Using articulating paper, identify the contacts and reduce lightly.

24. Repeat the procedure until simultaneous contact is achieved.

25. Check the ICP contacts to ensure that they have been maintained throughout the procedure.

26. Valve-grinding paste may be used to smooth small interferences, creating smooth lateral and protrusive movements.

27. Apply a thin layer of the paste to the occlusal surfaces of the teeth.

28. Move the articulator through the excursive pathways and make clockwise and anti-clockwise movements with the teeth in contact. The movements should feel smooth and free.

29. Carefully remove the dentures from the models using a plaster knife.

30. Wash off the grinding paste and place the dentures in an ultrasonic cleaner using a plaster solvent solution to remove any remaining plaster or stone.

31. Trim the flash using a large tungsten bur to restore the shape of the polished surfaces. The acrylic may be smoothed using stone or silicone burs, or sandpaper. Care should be taken to

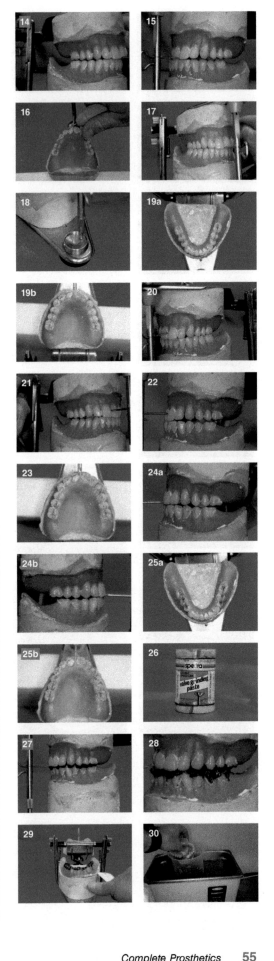

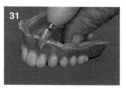
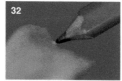

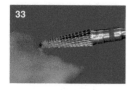
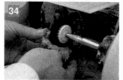

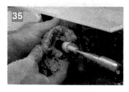
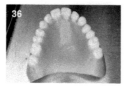

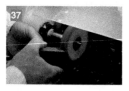
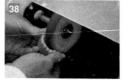

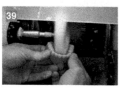
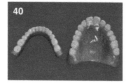

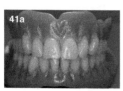
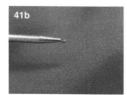

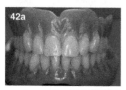
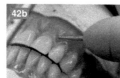

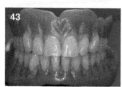
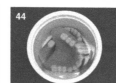

avoid grinding of the fitting surfaces or teeth during this procedure.

32. Inspect the fitting surface of the denture carefully to identify any blips caused by air bubbles in the surface of the model.

33. Remove these carefully using a fine tungsten bur.

34. Polish the surface of the denture using pumice and a brush on the polishing lathe. Pumice is mixed with water and used as a slurry. This helps to keep the pumice particles in contact with the acrylic and helps prevent burning of the acrylic. The pumice is an abrasive medium that removes the surface layer of the acrylic; thus, care should be taken to avoid removing any detail that has been carved into the surface of the dentures.

35. A variety of brush sizes and shapes are available for intricate areas.

36. The surface of the denture should be free from scratches prior to the polishing stage.

37. Tripoli (a polishing wax) is used with a cotton mop to polish the dentures.

38. Again a variety of brush sizes are available for hard to reach areas.

39. The dentures are buffed to a high polish using a soft wool mop.

40. The polished dentures should have a high gloss and be free from scratches.

41. The anterior labial surfaces of the dentures may be stippled using a stippling bur.

42. Move the bur in a circular motion over the surface at a slow speed.

43. The surface may require a light polish following this procedure.

44. Place the finished dentures into clean, cold water for 48 hours before they are fitted.

Extended information

The BULL rule

In a *normal arrangement* of the posterior teeth the following will apply:
In centric occlusion the buccal cusps of the mandibular teeth contact the central fossae of the maxillary teeth and the palatal cusps of the maxillary teeth contact the central fossae of the mandibular teeth. When making

Continued over

adjustments during lateral excursions only the buccal cusps of the maxillary teeth and the lingual cusps of the mandibular teeth (Buccal Upper and Lingual Lower) should be ground so as to maintain the mandibular buccal and maxillary palatal tooth contacts in centric.

If the posterior teeth have been set in a *cross-bite* the following will apply:

In centric occlusion the buccal cusps of the maxillary teeth contact the central fossae of the mandibular teeth and the lingual cusps of the mandibular teeth contact the central fossae of the maxillary teeth. When making adjustments during lateral excursions only the maxillary palatal and the mandibular buccal cusps should be ground to maintain the maxillary buccal and mandibular palatal contacts in centric. (This is the reverse of the normal BULL rule).

2.10 Denture repair

Denture repair   Single tooth repair

Introduction

Fractured dentures are common and relatively simple to repair (Figure 2.10.1). Read the extended information to ensure that you know whether a denture is worth repairing.

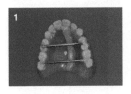

Figure 2.10.1

You will need:

- Sticky wax/model cement
- Denture wax
- Match sticks or old metal burs
- Wax carver/knife
- Tungsten carbide burs

- Anti-expansion solution and plaster of Paris
- Self-curing acrylic resin
- Water pressure bath/hydro-flask
- Polishing compounds and pumice

Work safety

Self-curing acrylic resin should be handled in a fume cupboard, wearing gloves. Grinding acrylic resin can also be dangerous, and eye protection and facemask must be worn and dust extraction used.

Basic procedure (fracture repair)

1. Assemble the broken pieces of denture carefully and secure with sticky wax. It may be necessary to strengthen the joint by securing an old bur across the teeth with sticky wax. On the fitting surface, block out with wax any large undercuts that do not involve the fracture site to enable easy removal of the model later.

2. Cast a model to the fitting surface of the denture using plaster mixed with anti-expansion solution; alternatively, use a silicone putty.

Continued over

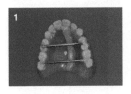
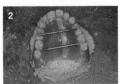

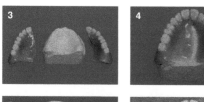

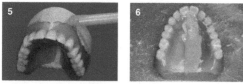

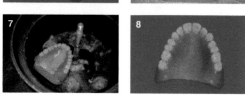

3. When set, remove the denture from the new model, and then remove the wax from the denture.

4. Reduce the broken ends slightly to expose clean acrylic resin, and create a definite gap between the two parts of the denture when assembled on the model. A finishing line for the repair resin to 'butt' up to can also be ground into the resin.

5. Paint the model with separating medium, position the denture on the model and secure with sticky wax.

6. Mix the acrylic and fill the gap, leaving a slight excess.

7. Place in a water pressure bath and cure for 15 minutes at 3 atm of pressure at 45°C.

8. After curing and removal of the denture from the model trim the cured material to leave the original contour of the denture.

9. Smooth with sandpaper and polish as described in Section 2.9.

Basic procedure (single tooth repair)

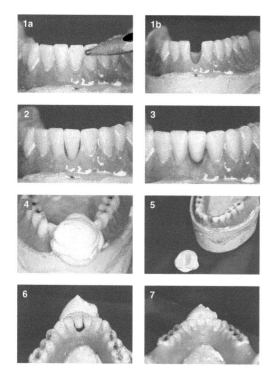

Fracture of a single tooth may involve the entire tooth or just a part of it may fracture, leaving a fragment attached to the denture base. If the entire tooth has come off the denture, this is usually due to poor bonding with the acrylic resin (usually caused by separating medium left on the tooth during processing). If the tooth has fractured and a part of the tooth left bonded to the denture base, there may be a problem with the occlusion and this should be checked and corrected after placing the new tooth.

In the following example a lower incisor was damaged during the processing of a denture.

1. Using a tungsten bur, remove the tooth from the denture.

2. Enlarge the tooth socket to allow room for new acrylic.

3. Position the new tooth in place using wax.

4. Mix a small amount of plaster using anti-expansion solution and make a plaster key to fit around the tooth, wax work and adjacent teeth and allow to set. Alternatively, use silicone putty.

5. Boil off the wax from the denture and plaster key.

6. Assemble the parts and secure with sticky wax.

7. Mix a small amount of self-curing acrylic to a runny consistency and fill the void. Place in a water pressure bath and cure for 15 minutes at 3 atm of pressure at 45°C.

8. Remove the plaster key and trim the denture to its original contour.

9. Polish the repair as described in Section 2.9.

Extended information

Midline fractures of the palate may be due to inadequate thickness of material, poor fit or unbalanced occlusion, in which case repair would be futile unless the cause of the fracture was identified and corrected.

Similarly in fractures originating from a structural defect such as a well-defined fraenal notch or a non-bonded tooth, the denture will fracture again unless the cause can be eliminated.

The incidence of fracture can be reduced by attention to the following points:

- Ensure that relief of fraenal attachments is not in the form of a sharp notch.

- Ensure that all acrylic teeth are free of contaminants before processing so that optimum bonding occurs between the teeth and the base.

- Ensure that dentures are adequately thick in cross-section.

There are a few useful methods for improving the strength of conventional polymethyl methacrylate dentures. Those in use are as follows.

Inserted materials

Inclusions such as stainless steel mesh or Nylon fabric decrease the strength as they do not bond to the acrylic and merely serve to keep the fractured ends in apposition until the 'strengtheners' themselves fail.

Inclusions which can bond to the resin will add considerable strength but have the disadvantage that they cause irritation to the mucosa if the fibres are exposed on the surface during polishing, which is almost inevitable. Some also have poor appearance (carbon fibre).

High-impact resins

High-impact resins incorporate rubber beads in the acrylic matrix that serve to interrupt crack propagation and prevent fatigue fracture. They are indicated when an elderly person habitually drops and breaks the dentures.

Alternative base materials

Cobalt–chromium is cast to fit the model accurately. Whilst mechanical locking between the metal and acrylic by means of meshwork is normal, both warrant the additional use of a 4-methacryloxy-ethyl trimellitate anhydride (4-META) resin to ensure good bonding between the metal base and the acrylic superstructure.

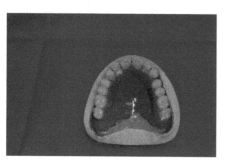

Figure 2.11.1

Introduction

Relining a denture is a means of creating a new fitting surface on an existing denture. This may be prescribed when the alveolar bone has resorbed, resulting in a poor fit and lack of retention (Figure 2.11.1).

Work safety

- Self-curing acrylic resin: Mix in a fume cupboard, wear gloves and wash your hands after use.
- Grinding acrylic resin: Wear eye protection and facemask, and use dust extraction.

You will need:

- Self-curing acrylic resin, mixing vessel and mixing spatula
- Plaster of Paris and dental stone
- Plaster bowl, spatula, plaster knife and mixing bowl
- Plaster-separating solution
- Tungsten carbide burs, sandpaper mandrel and sandpaper
- Temperature controlled water pressure bath or hydro-flask
- Strong elastic bands

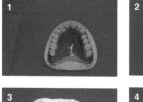
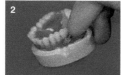
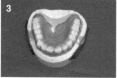
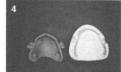
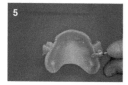
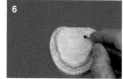
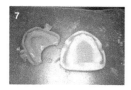
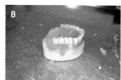

Basic procedure

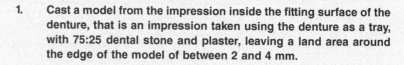

1. Cast a model from the impression inside the fitting surface of the denture, that is an impression taken using the denture as a tray, with 75:25 dental stone and plaster, leaving a land area around the edge of the model of between 2 and 4 mm.

2. Cut two 'V'-shaped notches in the land area, one on either side in the molar region, to a depth just short of the sulcus.

3. Coat the notches and surrounding area of the model with plaster-separating solution, then fill the notches with self-curing resin and allow to set and bond to the denture. This is to allow the relationship between the denture and the model to be maintained after the impression material has been removed.

4. Remove the denture from the model and clean the impression material from the fitting surface.

5. Roughen the fitting surface with a bur to aid the bonding of new acrylic material to the old. Create a finishing edge in the periphery of the denture to enable the new material to join smoothly to the old.

6. Cut a new post dam into the model.

7. Paint the model with plaster-separating solution, then mix the self-curing acrylic and spread over the fitting surface of the denture and model.

Continued over

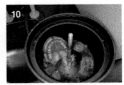

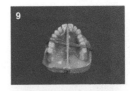

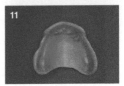

8. Replace the denture back on the model with the 'V'-shaped extensions locating fully into the notches to relocate the denture precisely back onto the model.

9. Place strong elastic bands around the denture and model to hold it in place during curing.

10. Place in a pressurised water bath or hydro-flask for 15 minutes at 45°C under 3 atm (40 psi) of pressure.

11. After curing, trim the excess acrylic resin, smooth, polish and store in clean cold water until required.

Extended information

The expected mean life of an unmodified denture is 4–5 years but the actual life depends on the rate at which alveolar resorption is taking place. Alveolar resorption is most significant when the teeth are first extracted, and some patients experience more alveolar resorption than others.

Indications for relining are as follows:

- Ridge resorption causing lack of retention with no deterioration of the polished or occlusal surfaces

- When a patient has difficulties adapting to a new denture

- As preliminary treatment (e.g. to restore the face height) before new dentures are made

- As a temporary measure to maintain the function of an immediate denture.

Clinical technique for a maxillary denture

1. All undercuts are removed from the fitting surface of the denture. This allows the denture to be removed from the model at the laboratory stage.

2. Holes are cut in the palate with a number 6 round bur to allow easy flow of the impression material from this region. A thin layer of impression a material is desired to avoid increasing the face height or altering the occlusal plane.

3. Any restoration of the periphery is made with green-stick impression compound or a functional extension material.

4. A new impression is taken in the fitting surface of the denture using either zinc oxide eugenol paste or silicone impression materials.

Continued over

Continued over

Hints and tips

To use heat-cured acrylic: invest the denture in plaster and dental stone in a two-part flask. Separate the parts and remove the impression material. Replace with heat-cure acrylic dough, close and cure as normal. Remember to roughen the surface of the old acrylic and prepare a finishing line for the new acrylic.

5. Coat the fitting surface with a fluid mix of impression material and take the impression with the opposing denture in place and contacting in the retruded position.

6. Muscle trim the periphery whilst the denture is kept under slight occlusal load.

Clinical technique for a mandibular denture

1. Mandibular alveolar resorption often results in loss of face height, which allows the impression to be taken without reduction to the fitting surface.

2. Remove all undercuts from the fitting surface as before.

3. Restore the periphery with green-stick impression compound or a functional extension material as necessary. Any necessary increase in face height is made at this stage.

4. Coat the fitting surface with impression material, take the impression with the maxillary denture in place and encourage the patient to close in RCP. Muscle trim the periphery whilst the denture is kept under slight occlusal load.

Existing denture | Impression taking | Copy denture technique

2.12 Copy dentures

Introduction

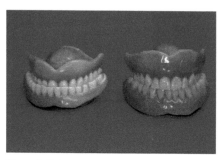

Figure 2.12.1

The aim of a copy denture technique is to transfer the contours of the old denture to the new. This helps the patient maintain control of the denture with the orofacial muscles and can be particularly helpful for older patients who have worn their dentures for a long time and would find habituating to a new denture shape difficult. The shape of the denture is conserved with only minor alterations for loss of fit (requiring an impression and change of fitting surface), increase in vertical dimension to reduce over-closure and replacement of worn teeth (Figure 2.12.1). Copy dentures are used to

• provide a spare set of dentures;

• produce new dentures with improved fitting surfaces, occlusal surfaces and vertical dimension whilst maintaining the shape;

• produce temporary dentures that can be modified gradually if the patient's ability to adapt to new dentures is in doubt.

There are numerous methods employed to carry out this procedure but all achieve the same outcome. First, a mould of the old denture is produced. Then a copy is produced that is adjusted as required, and the adjusted copy is processed into a new denture.

You will need:

- Impression material
- Two-part duplicating flask or any two-part containers which fasten together accurately, that is, a soap dish/holder
- Wax melting bath and wax – blue inlay wax provides a nice contrast to the pink denture base
- Self-curing acrylic resin
- Hydro-flask or warm water pressure bath
- Tungsten carbide burs, sandpaper mandrel, sandpaper articulator
- Plaster of Paris and dental stone plaster bowl
- Spatula and plaster knife
- Denture-processing flasks and clamp
- Acrylic resin curing bath
- Small round grinding stone
- Polishing unit, brushes, mops and polishing compounds and pumice

Basic procedure

1. Use a two-part flask to create a mould of the denture.

2. Fill one half of the flask and the fitting surface of the denture with alginate.

3. Place the denture in the flask such that the periphery of the denture is just covered. Trim excess impression material away level with the edge of the flask.

4. Once the material has set, coat with a thin layer of Vaseline.

5. Fill the other half of the flask with alginate and wipe material around the denture teeth and the polished surfaces with your fingers.

6. Place the two halves of the flask together and secure. The excess material will squeeze out from between the two halves and from the exit holes in the top.

7. Once set, open and remove the denture carefully. This may then be cleaned and returned to the patient.

8. Pour molten wax into the impression of the teeth and allowed to cool. This provides an exact copy of the denture teeth that will be easy to cut off and replace with new denture teeth.

9. Mix self-curing resin and pour into both halves of the flask.

10. Close the flask and secure with elastic bands.

11. Place into a water pressure bath to cure.

12. After 10 minutes, open the flask and remove the duplicate denture.

13. Use a tungsten carbide bur to trim away the flash.

Continued over

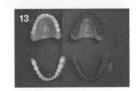
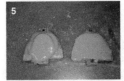
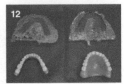
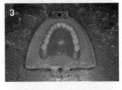
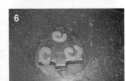
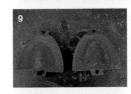
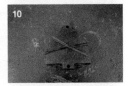
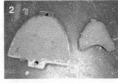
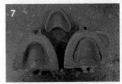
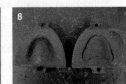
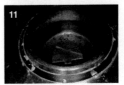
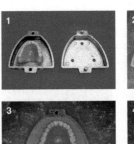
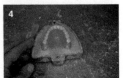

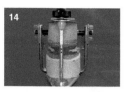
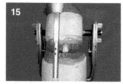
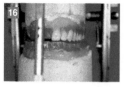
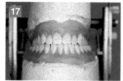
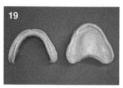
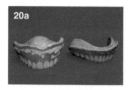
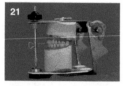
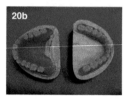
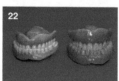

14. Mount the copy dentures on an articulator using the bite registration, and set to the correct vertical dimension.

15. Cut off the wax teeth one at a time and replace with the new acrylic teeth.

16. Start with the maxillary anterior teeth, then the maxillary posterior teeth and finally the mandibular posterior and anterior teeth as described in Section 2.7.

17. Check the occlusion of the posterior teeth, appearance of the anterior teeth and the wax work around the teeth. Take particular care not to alter the original contour of the dentures at this stage.

18. Return the dentures to the surgery for try-in.

19. After the try-in and checks for occlusal stability and appearance (any occlusal problems are dealt with by carrying out a re-try as normal) a corrective impression is taken inside the denture bases, usually in zinc oxide and eugenol impression paste (light- to medium-bodied silicones can also be used).

20. Cast working models to the impression inside the bases of the dentures.

21. Mount the models onto an articulator.

22. Process the dentures as described in Sections 2.8 and 2.9.

Hints and tips

Use a contrasting coloured wax for the impression of teeth to enable the demarcation between denture base and teeth to be seen.

Purpose-made duplicating flasks are available for copying dentures; these tend to be more accurate.

Extended information

Indications

- Dentures that have been worn satisfactorily for a long period of time may become ill-fitting as alveolar resorption takes place.

- Elderly and/or infirm patients who have difficulty learning to control new dentures.

Copy dentures only require the patient to attend the surgery on three to four occasions instead of the five to six visits for conventional new dentures. This is also a very convenient technique to use on domiciliary visits to patients who cannot get to the surgery. Copy dentures have their fit and occlusal relationships corrected but there is no alteration of the polished surface contour compared with the patient's original dentures. The patient should adapt to these dentures much more easily than they would to new conventional dentures.

Chapter 3 | PARTIAL PROSTHETICS

3.1 Introduction to partial prosthetics

Removable partial dentures are appliances that can be removed by the patient, and replace one or more missing teeth but not an entire arch.

A partial denture should

- restore appearance and masticatory function;
- be well retained and stable during function;
- be comfortable to wear;
- distribute occlusal forces favourably;
- prevent teeth drifting or over-erupting into edentulous spaces.

Partial dentures may be designed to utilise the remaining natural teeth in two ways. Firstly, the teeth can be used to aid the retention of the denture, keeping the denture in position. Secondly, the teeth may also be used to support the denture, distributing the occlusal forces applied to the denture through the hard tooth structure to the underlying bone.

The support for the partial denture may be considered and categorised as

- mucosa-borne (like a full denture), where support is gained from the underlying soft tissue (Figure 3.1.1);
- tooth-borne, where the support is distributed through the remaining natural teeth (Figure 3.1.2);
- tooth and mucosa-borne, where the support is provided by combination of the teeth and mucosa (Figure 3.1.3).

In this chapter, we discuss the classification, component parts, designing dentures, denture support (mucosa- and tooth-borne dentures) and the production of mucosa-borne and tooth-borne dentures.

3.2 Classification

Kennedy classification

This classifies the pattern of tooth loss in the order of frequency with which they are met in clinical practice.

Class I: Loss of the distal teeth bilaterally; any denture provided will have two free-end saddles (Figure 3.2.1). (A saddle is the tooth-bearing part of the denture.

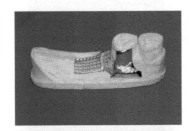

Figure 3.1.1

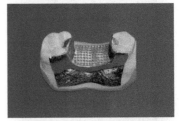

Figure 3.1.2

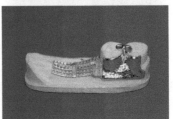

Figure 3.1.3

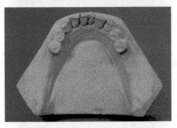

Figure 3.2.1

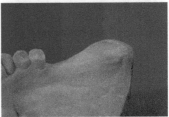

Figure 3.2.2

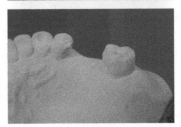

Figure 3.2.3

Basics of Dental Technology: A Step By Step Approach, Second Edition.
Tony Johnson, David G. Patrick, Christopher W. Stokes, David G. Wildgoose and Duncan J. Wood.
© 2016 John Wiley & Sons, Ltd. Published 2016 by John Wiley & Sons, Ltd.
Companion Website: www.wiley.com/go/johnson/basicsdentaltechnology

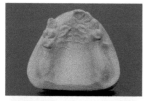

Figure 3.2.4

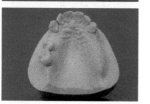

Figure 3.2.5

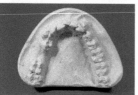

Figure 3.2.6

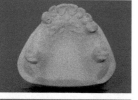

Figure 3.2.7

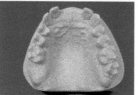

Figure 3.2.8

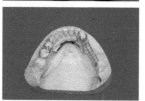

Figure 3.2.9

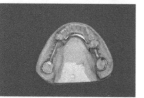

Figure 3.3.1

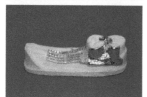

Figure 3.3.2

Figure 3.3.3

A free-end saddle has a no natural tooth at one end (Figure 3.2.2), whereas a bounded saddle is an edentulous area with natural teeth mesially and distally (Figure 3.2.3).)

Modifications can be added to this class when further teeth are lost creating extra bounded saddles; for example, Class I, modification 1, which has one extra bounded saddle (Figure 3.2.4).

Class II: Loss of the distal teeth unilaterally, requiring a denture with a single free-end saddle (Figure 3.2.5).

Modifications, involving extra bounded saddles, can be added as for Class I (Figure 3.2.6).

Class III: Loss of teeth producing a posterior bounded saddle (Figure 3.2.7).

Modifications can be added as in Classes I and II (Figure 3.2.8).

Class IV: Tooth loss producing an anterior bounded saddle (Figure 3.2.9).

No modifications are possible for this classification as the anterior saddle would become a modification of one of the other classes.

3.3 Component parts of partial dentures

Partial dentures have five distinct components: saddles, rests, clasps, reciprocation, and connectors.

Saddles

The saddle is the part of the denture that carries the artificial teeth over the edentulous area or saddle area. Saddles may be designed as mucosa-borne to transmit the occlusal load through the mucosa (Figure 3.3.1), or tooth-borne, where occlusal rests transmit the load to the adjacent teeth (Figure 3.3.2).

Saddles may be tooth- and mucosa-borne where the occlusal load is transmitted to both natural tooth and mucosa (Figure 3.3.3).

To minimise the load through the mucosa the extension of the saddle is designed to cover the maximum surface area possible, thus increasing the footprint of the saddle and spreading the load more widely. The occlusal table, (the surface area of the occlusal surface of the denture) may also be kept to a minimum by decreasing the bucco-lingual width of the denture teeth or by using less teeth.

Rests

Occlusal, incisal or cingulum rests are used to provide support for tooth-borne dentures by transmitting the occlusal load to the teeth (tooth-supported denture). They are small metal components that are an integral part of the denture base. This type of support prevents sinking of the denture (movement towards the mucosa) into the soft tissues by transferring occlusal loads to the remaining natural teeth. The natural teeth are prepared to have seats for the occlusal rests to prevent occlusal interference with the opposing teeth and to ensure that force is directed down the long axis of the tooth (Figures 3.3.4 and 3.3.5).

Rest seats should be saucer-shaped to allow good oral hygiene. If no occlusal interferences are likely, then rest seats need not be prepared.

Incisal and cingulum rests serve the same function on anterior teeth. Again, seats are prepared to prevent occlusal interference and avoid the unsightly appearance of metal at the front of the mouth. Rests on the lingual surface of canine teeth almost always require some preparation of the tooth, either to emphasise the cingulum or prevent interference with the opposing teeth.

Clasps (direct retainers)

Clasps provide retention (direct retention) for the denture. When fully seated, partial dentures are passive in the mouth. It is only when forces (sticky food) attempt to dislodge them that retentive elements become active. The flexible tip of a clasp arm contacts the tooth in an undercut area, remaining passive when seated, but exerting force when the denture is being removed.

There are two main types of clasp:

- Occlusally approaching (suprabulge): Approaches the undercut from the occlusal surface of the tooth. The entire arm contacts the tooth, but only the flexible tip enters the undercut to serve as the retainer (Figure 3.3.6).
- Gingivally approaching (infrabulge): Approaches the undercut from the gingival area and should only contact the tooth with the clasp tip (Figure 3.3.7).

Each type has several different designs and is discussed later in the chapter.

Reciprocation

When a clasp applies force to a tooth, some of that force acts laterally. This unfavourable force may lead to tooth movements or simply render the clasp inefficient. Therefore, reciprocation to this force is provided. This is a component that acts to maintain the tooth in position as the clasp exerts force. It lies on the opposite side of the tooth to the clasp tip and is either a reciprocating arm (Figure 3.3.8) or a plate (Figure 3.3.9).

Connectors

Connectors link the saddles and other component parts. They should be rigid, shaped such that they are comfortable for the patient, and hygienic, keeping distant from the gingival margin where possible.

Major connectors link saddle areas, and the most common are palatal plates (Figure 3.3.10) or bars (Figure 3.3.11).

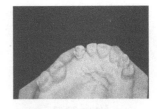

Figure 3.3.4

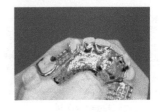

Figure 3.3.5

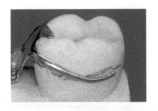

Figure 3.3.6

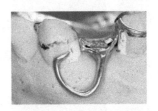

Figure 3.3.7

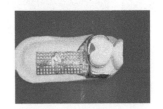

Figure 3.3.8

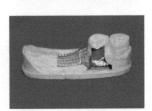

Figure 3.3.9

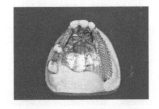

Figure 3.3.10

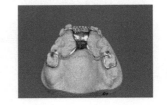

Figure 3.3.11

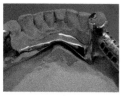

Figure 3.3.12

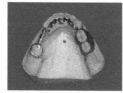

Figure 3.3.13

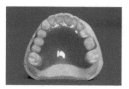

Figure 3.3.14

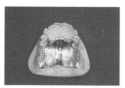

Figure 3.3.15

For mandibular dentures lingual bars (Figure 3.3.12) and plates are the most common (Figure 3.3.13).

Minor connectors attach small components such as occlusal rests and clasps to the denture. They should be designed to be hygienic and have the minimum bulk necessary while retaining adequate strength.

Denture base material

Partial denture bases are made of acrylic or cast cobalt–chromium. Acrylic is chosen for most mucosa-borne dentures and all temporary dentures (Figure 3.3.14). Cobalt–chromium alloy is used for tooth-supported designs, and occasionally for mucosa-borne dentures when indicated on account of its strength (Figure 3.3.15).

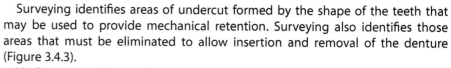

3.4 Surveying

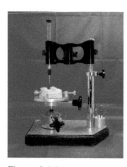

Figure 3.4.1

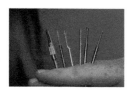

Figure 3.4.2

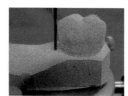

Figure 3.4.3

A surveyor is an instrument that is used to keep a tool in a parallel plane relative to a study model (Figure 3.4.1).

There are several tools that may be used in the surveyor arm (Figure 3.4.2):

- Graphite marker

- Analysing rod

- Chisel

- Measuring gauges

Surveying identifies areas of undercut formed by the shape of the teeth that may be used to provide mechanical retention. Surveying also identifies those areas that must be eliminated to allow insertion and removal of the denture (Figure 3.4.3).

Undercut may be used to create mechanical retention in two ways: firstly, by creating a path of insertion that is different to the path of displacement; and secondly, by engaging undercut with clasp arms (see Section 3.5).

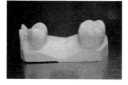

Figure 3.4.4

Creating a path of insertion

Consider the bounded saddle in Figure 3.4.4. Undercuts are easily identified to the mesial of the molar and the distal of the premolar (Figures 3.4.5 and 3.4.6).

This is undercut relative to the ***path of displacement***. The path of displacement is the pathway that the saddle will take when being dislodged by sticky food. We can assume that it is at right angles to the occlusal plane. There are five possible ways to produce a saddle in this situation:

1. Fill both undercut areas with the denture saddle (Figure 3.4.7)

The undercut areas relative to the path of displacement are both filled. This results in the saddle having excellent retention relative to the path of displacement; unfortunately, the denture cannot be withdrawn or inserted, making this unworkable.

2. Do no fill either of the undercuts with the denture saddle (Figure 3.4.8)

The undercut areas have been identified and 'blocked out' with plaster on the working model. The denture has been produced on the blocked out model; here,

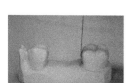

Figure 3.4.5

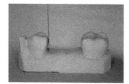

Figure 3.4.6

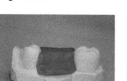

Figure 3.4.7

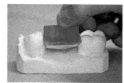

Figure 3.4.8

the undercut is not used and therefore no retention is gained. The path of insertion = path of displacement.

3. Fill the undercut mesial to the molar with the denture saddle (Figures 3.4.9 and 3.4.10)

The undercuts relative to the path of insertion are identified, and one is filled with the saddle to aid retention. To ensure that the denture may be removed, the undercut is blocked out distal to the premolar. Note that the plaster is angled to match the mesial surface of the molar, creating a path of insertion. The path of insertion is different from the path of displacement, creating retention.

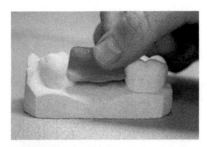

Figure 3.4.9

4. Fill the undercut distal to the premolar with the denture saddle (Figure 3.4.11)

5. Utilise the undercut distal to the premolar for retention

The final option is to utilise the undercut distal to the premolar for retention. The undercut mesial to the molar is eliminated and shaped to match that of the distal surface of the premolar. The path of insertion is different from the path of displacement creating retention (Figure 3.4.12).

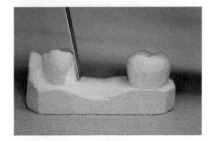

Figure 3.4.10

To aid the identification of these small undercut areas, a surveyor is used to hold the model on a horizontal platform. The vertical column allows tools to be moved around the teeth while maintaining the same plane.

Surveying to create a path of insertion

Previously, the surveying principle has been considered in relation to a single saddle. In practice, a patient may have two or three saddle areas with teeth adjacent to each. Here, the most favourable path of insertion should be sought.

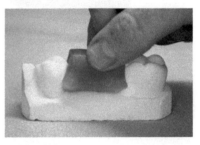

Figure 3.4.11

Displacement of a denture is often caused by the adhesion of food to the occlusal surfaces. This results in the displacement of the dentures at right angles to the occlusal plane. Therefore, creating a path of insertion that differs from the path of displacement improves retention.

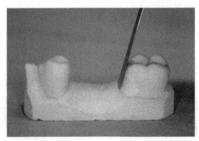

Figure 3.4.12

Basic procedure

1. Place the model on the surveyor table and secure.

2. Survey the model relative to the path of displacement, that is, with the occlusal plane at right angles to the analysing rod. Look for undercut areas relative to the path of displacement by holding the surveyor tool against the tooth. If no undercuts are found when surveying in this plane, mechanical retention cannot be used. Retention must be gained through physical and muscular forces.

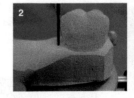
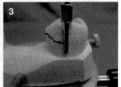

3. Using the graphite marker. Mark the survey line at this stage. This is the most bulbous part of the tooth.

Continued over

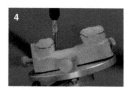

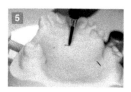

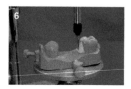

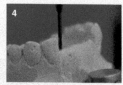

4. To use undercuts identified relative to the path of displacement, tilt the model on the surveyor such that the analysing rod is in line with the desired path of insertion, that is, tilt the model so the analysing rod can enter and contact the undercut you wish to use. Be sure that you are creating the best path of insertion for all saddle areas.

5. This position is now recorded to enable the model to be removed and replaced as necessary. To record this position, place the analysing rod against the side of the model on either side of the model and the back edge and draw a line against the model along the side of the analysing rod. Alternatively, set the height of the graphite mark and make three marks on the model.

6. The unwanted undercut is now eliminated by blocking out with plaster. This prevents the denture inadvertently being made to fill the undercut.

7. In most cases, the cast is now duplicated. This allows the denture to be produced on the duplicate and refitted to the original cast once complete.

Clasps should also be taken into consideration at this stage. See Section 3.5.

Hints and tips

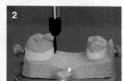

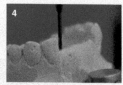

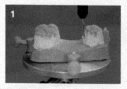

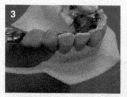

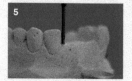

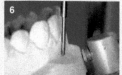

It is not always necessary or indeed possible to create a path of insertion that is different from the path of displacement. Often undercuts relative to the path of displacement are found and blocked out and a denture produced (1, 2).

Creating a path of insertion is aided by the provision of guide planes. These are flat surfaces that are cut into the natural tooth by the clinician. In the following examples, making the path of insertion different from the path of displacement would be an advantage and is simple to achieve.

1. *Bilateral free-end saddles* (3): The teeth naturally have undercuts on their distal surfaces. Here the model can be tilted to allow the denture to engage the undercuts. Any denture made to this path of insertion would in effect hook under this undercut, using it to resist vertical displacing forces.

2. *Anterior saddles* (4–6): Tilt the model to minimise undercuts on the mesial aspect of the abutment teeth.

This has the effect of eliminating unsightly gaps between the denture base and the teeth and helps prevent removal of the denture in a vertical direction by hooking into the undercuts mesial to the abutments.

The anterior saddle can also be surveyed to make the labial sulcus accessible and allow a flange to be placed.

Designing the partial denture is the responsibility of the clinician, although in practice the detail is often left to the technician. The disadvantage of this is that rest seats and guide planes that can be significant in the success of a denture tend to be overlooked. The design process should follow two phases.

1. The preparatory phase

This is undertaken to stabilise oral health. It includes prophylaxis and instruction in correct oral hygiene habits, motivation of the patient, removal of plaque-retaining factors, temporary restorations and removal of teeth that cannot be salvaged. It is often carried out with the help of a dental hygienist.

2. The corrective phase

The partly edentulous arch has often been damaged through incorrect loading. Restorative treatment may be necessary at this stage to correct significant problems with malaligned teeth or to improve the efficiency of the masticatory surfaces.

Adjustment of crown contour to aid denture design should be planned at this stage. This avoids inaccessible gaps, enhances support and retention by providing rest seats, additional undercuts and emphasising guide planes. Provision may also be made for minor connectors.

The design may be made and drawn on the study cast. The sequence below helps to ensure that all components are considered.

(1) Saddles: are identified and drawn on the cast.

(2) Survey: Undercuts are found relative to the path of displacement. These are either blocked out or a path of insertion created.

(3) Support: This is the resistance to displacing forces directed towards the mucosa. This is provided through mucosal coverage in the case of a mucosa-borne denture, through occlusal rests in tooth-borne dentures and a combination of the two in mucosa- and tooth-borne dentures.

(4) Retention: This is the resistance to force directed along the path of displacement. This can be provided by the physical and muscular forces in a similar way to complete dentures and may be enhanced by the addition of mechanical retention through creating a path of insertion or through clasping.

(5) Reciprocation: This ensures that clasps do not apply damaging forces to the teeth.

(6) Connectors: Join the other components together.

(7) Special techniques: Altered cast technique.

Designing saddles

Small edentulous areas should be left free from the denture design unless they are compromising aesthetics. Left free from denture components, small areas are self-cleansing and hygienic, but possible food traps if filled.

Mucosa-borne dentures should be designed to have the saddles cover the greatest surface area possible in order to distribute the load evenly and prevent

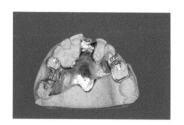

Figure 3.5.1

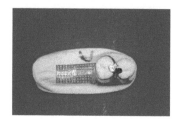

Figure 3.5.2

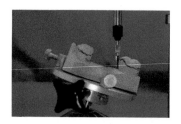

Figure 3.5.3

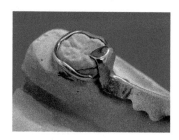

Figure 3.5.4

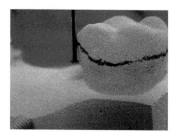

Figure 3.5.5

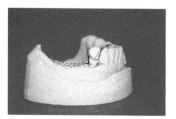

Figure 3.5.6

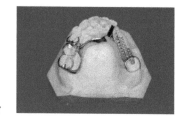

Figure 3.5.7

tissue damage. Reducing the occlusal table to the minimum necessary to oppose the natural teeth is also advantageous. Consider using narrower teeth that are more efficient at cutting through the food bolus and exert less pressure on the underlying tissue and ridge.

Design tooth-borne saddles to be hygienic and to harmonise with the natural teeth and soft tissues.

Be flexible in your choice of teeth. Space available for the replacement of a tooth is often reduced due to drifting of the remaining natural teeth; for example, consider using a premolar instead of a molar.

Designing tooth support

(1) Support for mucosal-borne dentures is provided by the fitting surface of the saddle area. Generally, the footprint of the denture should be as large as possible in order to gain maximum support.

(2) Tooth-borne dentures gain their support from occlusal rests positioned on teeth adjacent to the saddle area. Rests – occlusal, cingulum or incisal – transfer occlusal forces to the remaining teeth, reducing load on the saddle areas.

(3) Position rests for bounded saddles on the abutment teeth as near to the saddle area as possible (Figure 3.5.1).

(4) Ensure that they do not interfere with the occlusion. Rest seats should be prepared if the occlusion is likely to be compromised. Occlusal rests need to be at least 0.5 mm thick and should, preferably, be cast. Wrought rests can be used but tend not to fit as accurately as cast ones and are not as strong.

Designing tooth/mucosa support

(1) Position rests for free-end saddles (Class I and II) distant from the saddle area (Figure 3.5.2). This serves two purposes; first, it distributes the load to a tooth or a position on a tooth where the load can be opposed, and secondly, it can act as indirect retention (see section on indirect retention).

Designing retention

(1) Survey the teeth where clasping may be provided both buccally and lingually. If a path of insertion has been created, the teeth should be surveyed relative to the path of displacement and path of insertion (Figure 3.5.3).

(2) The clasp is designed such that the last third of the arm is positioned below the survey line (Figure 3.5.4).

(3) The position of the clasp tip is determined using a measuring gauge (Figure 3.5.5).

(4) A short, thick clasp arm will provide a very rigid clasp. This may be destructive to smaller teeth such as premolars. A thinner clasp is indicated in this situation (Figure 3.5.6).

(5) Conversely, long, thin clasp arms are flexible and unsuitable for molars as they would provide little retention (Figure 3.5.7).

(6) Check the occlusion when designing clasp arms that go over or between teeth; 2 mm clearance between the clasp arm and the opposing dentition is required. Tooth reduction or an alternative design should be considered if room is unavailable (Figure 3.5.8).

(7) Occlusally approaching clasps on the abutment teeth of free-end saddles should point towards the saddle (Figure 3.5.9). As the saddle moves along the path of displacement, the arm pointing towards the saddle is activated and helps to retain the saddle (Figure 3.5.10).

(8) A clasp pointing away from the saddle moves further into the undercut and does not aid retention (Figure 3.5.11).

(9) Gingivally approaching clasps tend to be more aesthetic when clasping canines and first premolars, as they are much less visible than occlusally approaching clasps (Figure 3.5.12).

(10) Reciprocation must be provided to oppose the action of each clasp tip.

Designing indirect retention

For free-ended saddles, clasping at the distal end is impossible. Indirect retention prevents the denture from rotating around the clasp tip as the saddle is displaced along the path of displacement. This is achieved by placing a rest (occlusal or cingulum) on the opposite side of the fulcrum (clasp tip) to the saddle area. The further away from the saddle they are, the more effective they are in forcing the clasp tip to move bodily up the tooth rather than rotating.

In the first two designs, no rest is provided (Figures 3.5.13 and 3.5.14). As the saddle is displaced, the clasp tip will engage the undercut and result in rotation of the denture.

The third design incorporates an occlusal rest mesially (Figure 3.5.15). This prevents rotation and forces the clasp to move bodily up the tooth rather than rotating on the spot.

Clasps designed in this way also benefit in that they disengage the undercut when under occlusal load.

Designing connectors

Connectors should be designed to be rigid, away from the gingival margins of teeth and cover as little tissue as possible. It is difficult to fulfil each of these requirements in each design as hygiene is compromised for strength and rigidity.

For mucosa-borne dentures

The denture is often made from acrylic only, and therefore, the strength of the connector must be gained through the bulk of material. The connector provides support and retention for the denture and therefore is made to cover much of the denture-bearing area (Figure 3.5.16).

Lingual bars may be produced in either cast or wrought metal for strength. They should be sited clear of the gingival margin and halfway between the teeth and the functional position of the floor of the mouth.

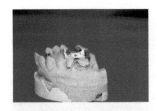

Figure 3.5.8

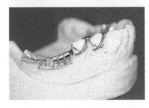

Figure 3.5.9

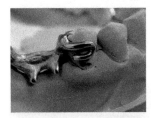

Figure 3.5.10

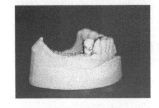

Figure 3.5.11

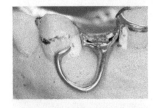

Figure 3.5.12

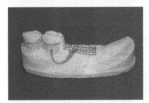

Figure 3.5.13

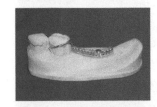

Figure 3.5.14

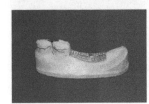

Figure 3.5.15

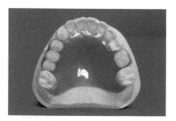

Figure 3.5.16

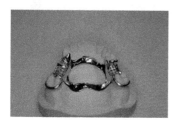

Figure 3.5.17

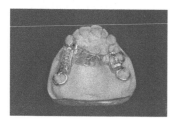

Figure 3.5.18

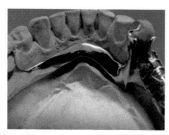

Figure 3.5.19

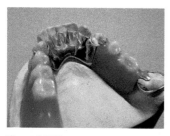

Figure 3.5.20

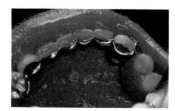

Figure 3.5.21

Lingual plates may also be produced in either acrylic or metal. Acrylic must be made thicker for adequate strength and may restrict tongue space. Metal plates are thinner, take up less space and can be highly polished to aid hygiene.

For tooth-borne dentures

The denture does not rely on the connector for support; therefore the framework may be kept to the minimum required for strength and rigidity (Figures 3.5.17 and 3.5.18). Plates are thinner than bars and are less likely to irritate the tongue, although the design is often dictated by patient preference.

Palatal plates should be as thin as possible and 'dammed' along the anterior and posterior borders to prevent food collecting beneath the denture. Palatal bars may be sited in the anterior, middle or posterior of the palate. The extent of the saddle areas is the determining factor. The middle bar is best tolerated by the tongue and soft palate.

Maxillary and mandibular connectors

Maxillary connectors are either plates or bars (Figures 3.5.17 and 3.5.18). In the mandibular arch, bars are used in preference to plates wherever possible to prevent covering the gingival sulcus and causing stagnation areas.

Lingual bars should be sited clear of the gingival margin and halfway between the teeth and the functional position of the floor of the mouth (Figure 3.5.19). They are contraindicated where there is insufficient space between the lingual sulcus and the gingival margins or when the lingual alveolus is markedly undercut. Lingually inclined teeth may also prevent their use.

Lingual plates can be made in thin section and are well tolerated (Figure 3.5.20). However, they do cover the gingival margins, contraindicating their use where oral hygiene is poor. Care must also be taken to avoid damage to the gingivae by providing appropriate relief during manufacture. A further problem occurs where there is pronounced gingival recession and anterior diastemas where the plate would be visible.

Sublingual bars are used in cases where space is restricted. They are designed to lie in contact with the floor of the mouth, which is recorded in the raised, functional position. They are indicated where there is little lingual gingival attachment and have the advantage of great rigidity.

The lingual bar and the continuous clasp (Kennedy bar) have the same cross-section as a lingual plate (Figure 3.5.21) with a hole cut to reveal the gingival margins. This connector can be irritating to the tongue.

A dental bar is used when there is insufficient room for a lingual or sublingual bar. It can also be used if the crowns of the teeth are long enough.

Labial and buccal bars and plates are used when there is marked lingual inclination of the teeth or the presence of excessive lingual undercuts. Manufactured in metal for strength, they are designed to be as thin and broad as the sulcus depth allows. They are produced on a relieved model to avoid direct tissue contact, but tend to interfere with the lip and cheeks. They are usually longer than lingual bars and should therefore have a greater cross-sectional area for rigidity.

Loss of teeth may lead to poor appearance, defects of speech chewing, over-eruption and rotation of opposing teeth, migration and tilting of adjacent teeth, food impaction, pocket formation and alveolar bone loss.

Current indications for denture provision vary a lot. This is due to the differences between patients' needs, requirements, desires and motivation towards maintaining their oral health.

The practice of replacing any missing tooth with a denture is contraindicated for several reasons. The World Health Organization recommends that a satisfactory dentition is one with 12 or more pairs of opposing teeth. New techniques, particularly adhesive bridges, and also the use of implants are less damaging to the remaining teeth, which has negated the use of some partial dentures.

Further, good oral hygiene instruction is a better prophylactic measure than a partial denture. Tooth loss following replacement of teeth with a partial denture is greater than when other methods of tooth replacement are employed. This may be attributed to the increased plaque accumulation that in turn leads to caries, gingivitis and periodontal disease.

With the exception of 'transitional' partial dentures, designed to make the path to complete dentures easier, only appearance and masticatory function remain as significant indications for partial denture provision.

A patient's main demand of a partial denture is good appearance and retention. Dentures replacing upper anterior teeth are well tolerated and used whereas those used for functional purposes only, replacing missing lower posterior teeth, are not. For this reason, in the absence of pressing indications, partial dentures should not be provided unless requested by the patient.

- The design should be as simple as possible to include the requirements for support, retention and strength.
- Permanent mandibular partial dentures should have a large footprint to prevent trauma to the soft tissues.
- Provision of a denture saddle posterior to a natural molar abutment is difficult to justify.
- Permanent lower partial dentures are best designed as a tooth-supported metal denture as there is limited soft tissue support available.
- Clear embrasure spaces are provided between saddles and abutments as well as a 3 mm gap between connectors and gingival margins to allow for self-cleansing.
- Special impression techniques (such as the altered cast technique) for mandibular free-end saddle partial dentures are highly recommended in order to provide a more comfortable and stable result during mastication.

3.6 Partial denture construction – acrylic resin

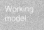

Working model → Blocking out → Manufacture of metal or acrylic denture base

Introduction

Acrylic resin partial dentures (Figure 3.6.1) are relatively simple appliances but are often poorly designed and constructed. They are often thought to be a temporary situation until complete tooth loss is reached. This is not necessarily the case, as good design and construction can provide a well-fitting, hygienic appliance.

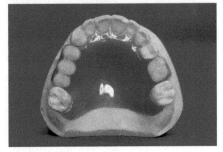

Figure 3.6.1

You will need:

- Dental stone (Kaffir D)
- Plaster of Paris
- Working model
- Wax knife
- Bunsen burner
- Laboratory silicone
- Light-curing acrylic resin blanks and light-curing box
- Denture wax
- Vaseline
- Plaster separating solution
- Acrylic resin
- Tungsten carbide burs
- Sandpaper mandrel and sandpaper

Work safety

Wear safety goggles and use dust extraction when trimming acrylic.

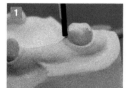

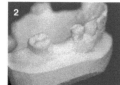

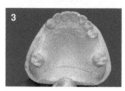

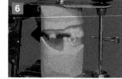

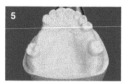

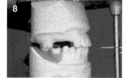

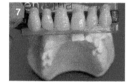

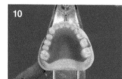

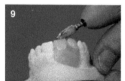

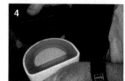

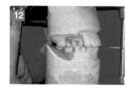

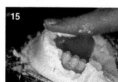

Basic procedure

Model construction

1. Place the model on the surveyor and survey relative to the path of displacement.

2. Block out undercuts mesial and distal to the saddle area with plaster or wax. Alternatively, create the path of insertion and block out the unwanted undercuts.

3. Cut a dam around the periphery of the denture design.

4. If using a duplicate model, create a mould of the working model in a duplicating flask using agar (see Section 3.7, stages 6–10); alternatively, take an impression using silicone in a stock tray.

5. Cast the duplicate model in a 25:75 plaster/Kaffir.

Setting up the denture teeth

6. Mount the models on an articulator using the occlusal record provided, Bonwill triangle and the split-cast mounting technique.

7. Choose teeth that match the size of the remaining natural teeth.

8. Set the teeth into the registration rim or create a baseplate using wax or light-cured acrylic.

9. Adjust anterior teeth to match the contours and wear facets on the adjacent natural teeth.

10. Check the occlusal contacts and adjust to conform with the natural teeth.

11. Use teeth that best fit the space; consider the use of two pre-molars when replacing one lost molar if the natural teeth have drifted and the gap has been reduced.

12. Contour the wax to match the natural gingivae.

Try-in of the wax denture

13. The normal stages of a try-in are carried out.

14. Ensure anterior teeth meet the patient's requirements.

Processing a heat-cured denture

Flask, pack and process the denture as described for complete dentures with the following modifications:

15. When flasking the model in the shallow half of the flask, cover the 'natural' teeth with plaster as shown.

Continued over

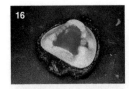
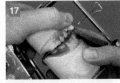
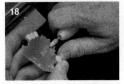
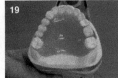

16. Smooth the plaster under running water. This allows the mould to be separated.

17. De-flask and remount the denture onto the articulator and adjust the occlusion.

18. Remove the denture from the model carefully, trimming away the plaster if necessary. Trim the acrylic and polish.

19. The denture may be fitted to the duplicate model if requested or adjusted at the chairside to fit.

Hints and tips

Acrylic resin partial dentures can be very weak compared with cobalt–chromium dentures and can fracture frequently. Inserting metal strengtheners, particularly in mandibular partial dentures, can considerably strengthen the denture.

If no clasps are present, adhesion will be a major retentive force so the denture should extend to cover the entire available denture-bearing area.

When anterior teeth are to be replaced it is important to ensure that the path of insertion and removal is such that no unsightly gaps are left between the denture and the natural teeth/tissues (undercuts) as aesthetics are likely to be the patient's main consideration. A secondary benefit of this is the added resistance to dislodging the forces that this alteration to the path of insertion and removal will create.

3.7 Partial denture construction – cobalt–chromium

Working model > Blocking out > Manufacture of metal or acrylic denture base

Introduction

Cobalt–chromium partial dentures are lighter and stronger because they cover less hard and soft tissues than acrylic resin partial dentures, and are more hygienic. However, poorly designed and constructed dentures can damage the remaining natural teeth. Care should be taken to ensure that wherever possible, the design and construction of these appliances does not cause damage to, or loss of, hard and soft tissues within the oral environment.

You will need:

As for acrylic resin partial denture, plus:

- Class IV die stone
- Plaster of Paris
- A master model and a duplicate master model
- Denture wax
- Reversible hydrocolloid + a temperature-controlled melting bath
- Beeswax or rosin + a temperature-controlled melting bath

- A drying oven
- Assorted wax profiles
- Silicone impression (after guide planes and rest seats prepared)
- Sprue wax; cone formers; plastic casting rings
- Phosphate-bonded investment material; pre-cast liquid investment
- Aluminium oxide 25–50 μm + sandblaster machine
- Carborundum cut-off discs; tungsten carbide burs; hard rubber wheels

Work safety

When using phosphate-bonded investment materials and grinding cobalt-chromium alloys always wear eye protection and a facemask and mix/grind using fume and particulate extraction.

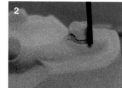
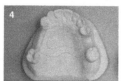
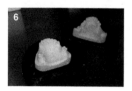
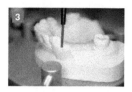
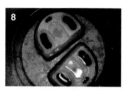
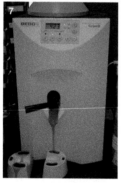
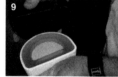
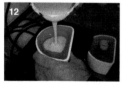
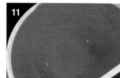
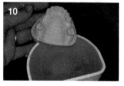
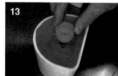
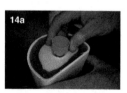
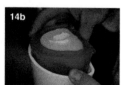
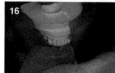
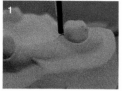
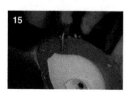

Basic procedure

Producing a wax pattern for casting

1. Cast the master model in class IV die stone to provide maximum resistance to abrasion during the construction process and position on the surveyor.

2. Survey the model and determine the path of insertion as described in Section 3.4.

3. Block out the unwanted undercut using plaster or blocking out wax.

4. Cut a dam around the periphery of the design and position 0.5 mm sheet wax over the saddle areas to provide relief for the framework. Note the relief wax in position where the gingivally approaching clasp is to be placed adjacent to the canine.

5. Duplicate the master model using agar to create a refractory (heat-proof) model. Here an upper and lower cast are being duplicated.

6. Soak the model in room-temperature water for 20 minutes and place it on the base of the duplicating flask.

7. Place the flask over the base and close firmly. Fill the flask with agar (maintained in a molten state in a thermostatically controlled bath).

8. When full, leave for 20 minutes while the agar initially sets, and then place in a bath of cool tap water to just below the top of the flask for a further 20 minutes.

9. Remove the base of the flask.

10. Carefully remove the model.

11. The fine detail of the model surface should be clear.

12. Pour a duplicate model using phosphate-bonded investment, mechanically mixed under vacuum and carefully vibrated into the mould. Leave for 1 hour to set before removing the duplicating material.

13. For lower models, a sprue former is inserted prior to pouring the investment.

14. Once set, remove the sprue former (if used) and remove the agar mould from the flask.

15. Taking care not to damage the model, section the agar.

16. Remove the sections.

Continued over

17. The agar can be rinsed with water and reused.

18. Heat the investment model in an oven to approximately 200°C to dry the model.

19. Dip into a heated bath of beeswax or rosin for 2–3 s.

20. Allow to cool and dry.

21. Survey the refractory model.

22. Mark the position of the clasp tips.

23. The wax pattern can now be laid onto the surface of the model. Components for wax patterns are supplied pre-formed: sheet wax of varying thicknesses, wax clasps in different sizes, wax retention sections in various shapes and sizes.

24. Press the wax pattern components into place following the design drawn.

25. Start by placing the retention wax over the relieved area.

26. Pre-formed clasps are available in various shapes and sizes, and curved for left or right teeth.

27. Position the clasp tip on the position marked.

28. Working around the tooth, adapt the wax arm along the survey line.

29. The thick end of the clasp should be cut to length such that it finishes in the saddle area.

30. Smaller clasps are chosen for the occlusally approaching clasp on the premolar.

31. Adapt this to the tooth, again positioning the clasp tip first.

32. Cut to length to finish in the saddle area.

33. Repeat the process for other occlusally approaching clasps.

34. Here, gingivally approaching 'T' clasps are being used.

35. Position the clasp tip and adapt the arm over the relieved area of the model to the saddle area.

36. Cut to length such that the arm joins the retention mesh wax. The clasp tip has been modified in this example to form an 'I' bar.

37. Join each component using modelling wax.

Continued over

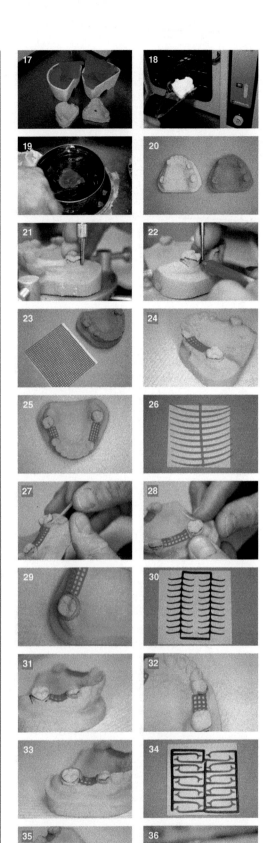

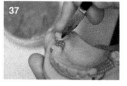
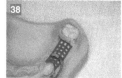

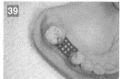
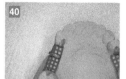

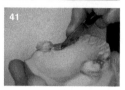
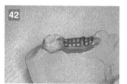

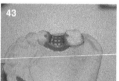
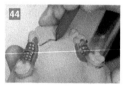

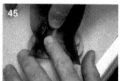
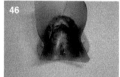

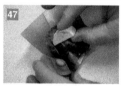
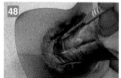

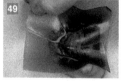
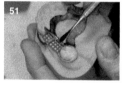

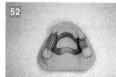
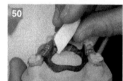

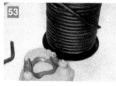
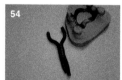

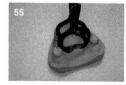
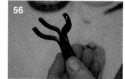

38. Fill the spaces in the retention wax adjacent to the gingivally approaching clasp. This will allow the molten casting alloy to flow readily into the mould.

39. Create the occlusal and cingulum rests by filling the rest seats with wax.

40. Carve the wax to make a smooth surface and ensure that the rest is attached to the clasp and retention wax.

41. Create a finishing edge for the acrylic using modelling wax or a length of wax profile.

42. Make a smooth transition between finishing edge, clasps and rests.

43. Repeat for all saddle areas.

44. Outline the peripheral dam using a pencil.

45. Adapt a sheet of wax to the model to form the connector. Warm the wax gently to soften if required.

46. To allow the wax sheet to adapt, cuts may be made to avoid stretching. Ensure that any folding that is necessary occurs outside the wax pattern.

47. Using your thumb or a rubber, adapt the wax until passive.

48. Using a scalpel, cut around the peripheral dam, leaving wax over the dam and to provide reciprocation to clasps where necessary.

49. Remove small sections of the excess wax at a time.

50. Once removed, ensure that the wax remains adherent to the model.

51. Blend the connector into the finishing edges.

52. The wax pattern is now ready for investing and casting.

Investing and casting the wax pattern

53. The wax pattern is sprued using 4 mm wax.

54. Join two lengths together to form a 'Y' shape as shown.

55. Adjust the width between the sprues such that they may be attached to the occlusal rests.

56. Repeat the process for the anterior rests and join all four sprues together.

Continued over

57. Attach the sprues to the occlusal rests using modelling wax. Ensure that the transition is smooth.

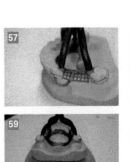

58. A split ring former is used to create the refractory mould.

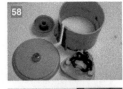

59. Secure the model to the ring base using sticky wax.

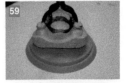

60. Using the ring former as a guide, adjust the length of the sprues such that a spruing cone can be positioned level with the plastic casting ring rim. This funnel should direct the alloy down the sprues and into the casting.

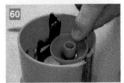

61. Seal the sprues to the cone.

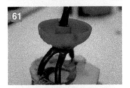

62. Ensure that the transition is smooth to minimise turbulence in the molten alloy.

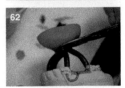

63. Coat the wax pattern with a thin layer of liquid investment to reduce surface tension on the wax and ensure a good adaptation of investment.

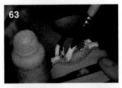

64. Assemble the ring former on the base.

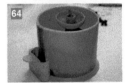

65. Vacuum mix the investment material and vibrate into the ring and around the wax pattern and model.

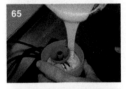

66. Once set (1 hour) remove the plastic casting ring former and heat the mould to 900–1000°C in a furnace to remove the wax and thermally expand the mould. Heat soak for 30 minutes.

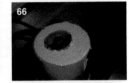

67. Heat the alloy, here in an induction casting machine.

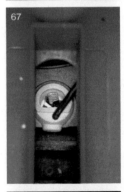

68. As the alloy approaches the casting temperature of approximately 1450°C stop heating (follow manufacturer's instructions).

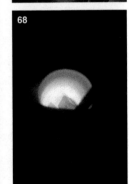

69. Remove the mould from the furnace and place in casting machine.

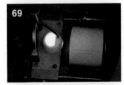

70. Heat alloy to casting temperature and cast into the mould.

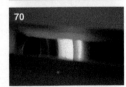

71. Remove from casting machine and allow to bench cool to room temperature.

72. Remove the investment using a small hammer.

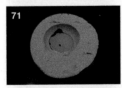

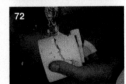

73. The refractory model is discarded with the investment material.

74. Repeatedly hit the button with a hammer to remove the remaining investment material. Pneumatic hammers are available for this.

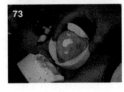

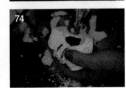

75. Clean the casting using a shot blaster.

Continued over

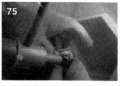
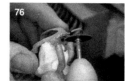

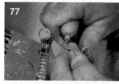
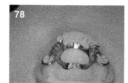

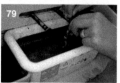
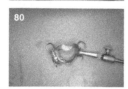

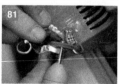
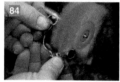

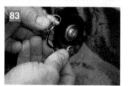
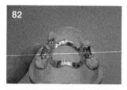

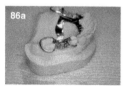
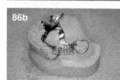

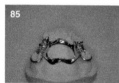

76. Cut the sprues from the casting using carborundum discs.

77. Trim the occlusal rests to shape and remove any casting defects with tungsten carbide burs.

78. Fit the framework to the original model. Take care to relieve the metal work where necessary to avoid damage to the model.

79. Attach the framework to the anode in an electrolytic polishing bath keeping the framework 4–5 cm away from an inert stainless steel cathode. The electrolyte solution should be 18–20°C. With an electric current of 12 V polish for 5 minutes; then remove and wash off the electrolyte under cold water; then polish again for a further 5 minutes.

80. Remove from the bath and rinse under cold water.

81. Remove scratches from the non-fitting surface with a rubber wheel.

82. The framework is now ready for a final polish.

83. Polish with hand-held bristle brushes and polishing compound and then complete the polish using a polishing lathe.

84. Buff with a cotton mop.

85. The framework should fit passively.

86. Return the framework to the clinician on the master model for a try-in.

Try-in of metal base

1. The base must fit accurately.

2. The occlusion of the natural teeth with the denture in place should be the same as without the denture.

3. Problems may occur with rests that have been made too thick or too high occlusally due to insufficiently deep rest seats.

4. Also connectors for occlusally approaching clasps that go over or between the natural teeth may interfere.

5. Interferences are detected using articulating paper.

6. Wax registration rims can be attached to the metal try-in at this stage to allow the registration to be carried out along with the metal try-in.

Setting of teeth and finishing processes are the same as for acrylic dentures.

Extended information

The mould is heated for three purposes: Firstly, to remove the wax from the mould; secondly, to prevent the molten alloy from freezing when filling the mould; finally, to expand the mould sufficiently to counteract the contraction of the cooling metal.

There are several different types and many makes of machine used to melt and cast cobalt–chromium alloy. The most widely used system is induction coil melting and centrifugal casting. Torch melting using oxy-acetylene can be used but tends to impart carbon into the alloy and make it brittle. An increasingly popular melting/casting method is the induction coil melting and pressure/vacuum casting system.

When producing a lower cobalt–chromium partial denture it is possible to attach the sprues to the wax pattern through the bottom of the model. A casting cone is placed into the agar duplicating mould prior to the investment being poured in to make the model. The cone creates a cone-shaped hole in the base of the model for the sprues to be attached.

Hints and tips

- Use round sprue profiles, as rectangular-shaped sprues can restrict the flow of alloy.
- Make the sprues thicker than any part of the casting and attach to the thickest part of the casting to ensure the mould fills completely. Thick sprues allow molten metal to be drawn into the casting as the alloy cools and contracts on cooling – the casting can draw molten alloy from the thicker sprue as this will cool last of all and thus acts as a reservoir.
- Follow the manufacturer's instructions rigidly using a matched alloy/investment combination to ensure the correct thermal expansion of the investment.
- Do not re-use the cobalt–chromium alloy. The beneficial properties of the base elements in the alloy, which help to produce a porous-free, strong casting, are expended on melting. Subsequent casting of the same alloy may be weaker and prone to porosity.

Chapter 4 | FIXED PROSTHODONTICS

Fixed prosthodontics includes indirect restorations that are produced in the laboratory and permanently fixed to the dentition. Depending on the area of the tooth to be covered or the shape of the preparation designed by the clinician, these are given different names: crown, inlay, onlay and three-quarters crown. These may be single units, or incorporated into a multi-unit bridge design.

- Full crown: Covers the entire clinical crown (Figure 4.1)
- Partial crown: Covers only portions of the clinical crown (Figure 4.2)
- Inlay: An intra-coronal restoration (Figure 4.3)
- Inlay: Occlusal inlay (Figure 4.4).

Each of these restorations can be further categorised depending on the material from which they are constructed:

- Metal (Figure 4.5)
- Metal-ceramic (Figure 4.6)
- All-ceramic (Figure 4.7).

One complication is that there are different processing or manufacturing routes for each of the materials that may also contribute to their names:

- Lost wax process
- Sintered
- Computer-aided design (CAD)–computer-aided manufacturing (CAM)
- Hot pressed
- Slip cast
- Laser sintered.

In this chapter, indirect restorations will be categorised using the material from which they are constructed, with further discussion of other processing routes in the Extended information box.

4.1 Restoration design

Marginal fit

Marginal fit is the degree of accuracy between the prepared tooth and restoration at the margin. The accuracy of fit should be around 25 μm although less than

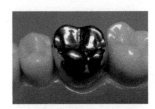

Figure 4.1

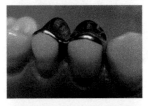

Figure 4.2

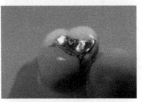

Figure 4.3

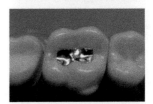

Figure 4.4

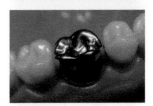

Figure 4.5

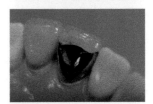

Figure 4.6

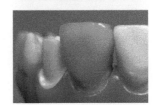

Figure 4.7

Basics of Dental Technology: A Step By Step Approach, Second Edition.
Tony Johnson, David G. Patrick, Christopher W. Stokes, David G. Wildgoose and Duncan J. Wood.
© 2016 John Wiley & Sons, Ltd. Published 2016 by John Wiley & Sons, Ltd.
Companion Website: www.wiley.com/go/johnson/basicsdentaltechnology

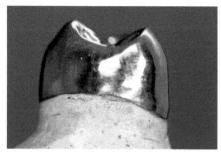

Figure 4.1.1

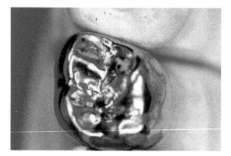

Figure 4.1.2

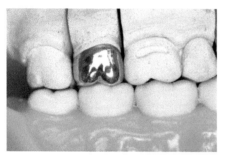

Figure 4.1.3

100 μm has been suggested as clinically acceptable. As a guide the diameter of an average human hair is around 40 μm.

Poor marginal fit may result in the need for additional treatment with the associated increase in time, cost or tooth loss (Figure 4.1.1).

Emergence angle

The emergence angle, or profile, is the angle at which the natural contour of a tooth appears to emerge from the gingival tissues. Where an emergence angle is made too acute, the surrounding gingiva may be displaced. Conversely, where the restoration surface is under contoured, a stagnation area (crevice at the gingival sulcus) is likely to result.

Contact points (contact areas)

The contact with the adjacent tooth prevents drifting and rotation, and is positioned just below the marginal ridge (about two-thirds of the way up the proximal surface) (Figure 4.1.2).

The contact point provides a gap, called an embrasure, which is open and should not encroach on the interdental papilla (Figure 4.1.3).

The embrasure is the area between adjacent surfaces as they flare away from one another, such as those found above and below the proximal contact area, or the space formed by the interproximal contours of adjoining teeth or restorations.

The surface is made convex to allow easy cleaning by the patient using dental floss.

Tooth contour

The shape of the restoration should have a natural contour, harmonising with the adjacent teeth. The bulbous shape of the tooth protects the delicate gingival sulcus during mastication.

Occlusion

Contact with the opposing teeth needs to be established to prevent over-eruption of the restored and opposing teeth.

Where a single crown or small anterior bridge is being constructed and the remaining teeth are intact, the models are usually held together by hand to check the occlusal contacts. Where extensive restorative work is being undertaken, the models should be articulated to allow repeated accurate positioning and movement to be achieved.

4.2 Metal restorations

All-metal restorations are extensively used in dentistry and their popularity may be attributed to their many advantages over the other types of restoration. Metal restorations, typically gold alloys, can be designed as full veneer crowns, inlays, onlays, three-quarter crowns, post crowns and bridges.

Advantages:

- Minimal tooth reduction in comparison to a porcelain-fused metal (PFM) or all-ceramic restoration, due to high strength of the material.

- Strong, robust, accurate and simple to produce.

- Margins are simple, hygienic, and some may be burnished for an improved marginal seal.

- Occlusal adjustment is simple and the alloys are easy to re-polish intra-orally.

- Convenient for rest seats, guide planes, reciprocal ledges and undercuts in conjunction with partial dentures. They may be soldered, and consequently can be joined to other metal structures or re-contoured, for example, to extend a short proximal contact.

- Wear characteristics are similar to enamel.

Disadvantages:

- Poor aesthetics, therefore limited to posterior restorations.

- Biocompatibility of all metals is an issue of ongoing debate.

Processing routes

The conventional processing route for metal restorations is the lost wax casting technique. Here, a wax pattern is produced, a heat-resistant mould is made around this, the wax is removed by melting and the resultant void is filled with molten metal.

CAD–CAM processing routes are available. One method is to design the restoration using computer software and to mill the pattern in a plastic material that can be invested in place of the conventional wax pattern. This has the advantage that the wax pattern production stage is eliminated and the plastic restoration may be tried in the patient's mouth prior to production in metal. It is also possible to 3D print a wax pattern from an electronic design. Alternatively, the restoration can be designed using computer software and sent electronically to an external processing company, where industrial technology is then used to laser sinter the alloy to produce the restoration. See section 4.25 for more information on Digital Dentistry.

Features of all-metal tooth preparations

Although all preparations for all-metal restorations are unique, they should follow the following principles to ensure adequate strength, retention and hygiene.

- Occlusal and axial reduction of 0.5 mm (the minimum casting thickness of gold).

- Convergence angle between 4° and 11° for retention and resistance for the restoration.

- Chamfered margin (marginal integrity).

- Undercuts must be avoided.

- Sharp external angles should be rounded to allow die material to flow into the fine detail and avoid air being trapped in the impression. This also prevents damage to the die during wax-up, or trapping of air during refractory pouring.

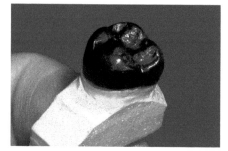
Figure 4.3.1

4.3 Ditching the die

Introduction

This procedure is carried out to enable the technician to access the margin of the preparation on the model. The soft tissue area around the prepared tooth on the working model is removed (Figure 4.3.1).

You will need:

- Sectioned model (see Sections 1.12 and 1.15)
- Round bur
- Scalpel
- Pencil

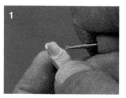
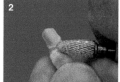
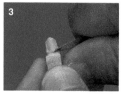
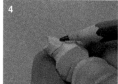

Basic procedure

1. Remove the die to be ditched from the model and identify the margin. Working from below the level of the margin, trim away the soft tissue until the bottom of the gingival pocket is reached.

2. You may need to do this in two stages, removing the bulk of the material first and repeating the process to remove the small remainder.

3. A scalpel may be used to remove very small amounts of material or when the tissue is close to the margin.

4. Continue around the die, and the result should be an exposed margin. Highlight this with a pencil.

4.4 Producing a wax pattern

Introduction

In preparation for metal casting, the restoration is made from wax on the working model (Figure 4.4.1).

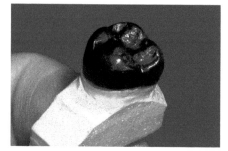
Figure 4.4.1

You will need:

- A ditched die on a sectional model
- Die hardener
- Die spacer
- An opposing model
- Wax knife, carver and Bunsen burner
- Tissue paper
- Separating medium
- Inlay wax
- Wax dipping pot (if available)
- Wax sheet

Basic procedure

1. Cover the die with a thin coat of die hardener and blow excess off immediately. There should be no residual material on the surface of the die.

2. Apply two coats of die spacer to allow room for the luting cement. This should finish 1 mm above the margin to ensure a tight marginal fit.

3. Once dry, apply separator to the die, adjacent and opposing teeth, using a brush.

4. Remove the excess using compressed air or a paper tissue.

5. Dip the die into the pot of molten wax until the margins are submerged.

6. Remove and allow to solidify. A drip always forms; this can be reduced by touching it on the rim of the pot, alternatively hold the die such that the drip will harden where extra wax is required, such as the tip of a cusp.

7. If using sheet casting wax, gently fold this around the preparation and join together.

8. Trim the wax back to the margin. Remove a band of wax up to 1 mm above the margin. Replace this with hard inlay wax if the wax contracts away from the margin.

9. By adding wax, extend the coping to form contact points with the adjacent teeth.

10. Ensure that the shape interproximally between the teeth does not encroach on the soft tissues. At this stage it is worth ensuring that the pattern can be removed and replaced on the die.

11. Add wax incrementally to build cusp tips.

12. Use the opposing model as a guide.

13. Add wax to the lingual and buccal aspects of the restoration so that when looking from above (occlusally) your pattern is in harmony with the adjacent teeth.

14. The occlusal surface should be modelled to represent the tooth morphology, taking into account the cuspal patterns on the surrounding dentition.

15. Ensure that the functional cusps are in contact with the opposing tooth.

16. The surface finish should be smoothed by gently abrading the wax with soft tissue.

17. Check the marginal fit, contact points, emergence profile, morphology, and surface finish.

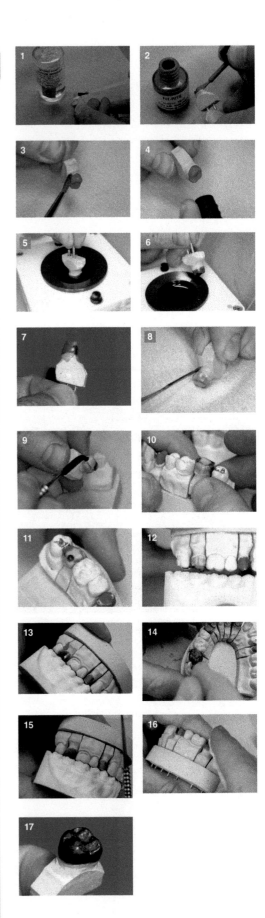

Wax pattern production > Investing > Casting and de-vesting

4.5   Investing the wax pattern

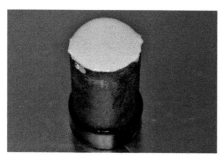

Figure 4.5.1

Introduction

A mould of the wax pattern is now made from a refractory material (Figure 4.5.1).

The objective is to mount the pattern at its thickest point such that it is positioned 3–5 mm from the end of the casting ring. Spruing at the thickest point of the pattern serves two functions: it acts as a channel for the molten metal to flow through, and as a reservoir of molten metal that the contracting casting can draw on during solidification. The pattern is positioned close to the end of the mould to allow the air within the mould to escape through porosities in the refractory material. This is necessary as the molten metal seals the mould on entry.

Basic procedure (for a single gold crown)

1. Cut a 5 cm length of 3 mm spruing wax. Soften one end and using fingers, lightly shape to a point.

2. Preserving as much morphology of the crown as possible, attach the pointed end of the sprue to the mesio-palatal (biggest) cusp. A small amount of sticky wax may be used if necessary.

3. Ensure the join between the sprue and crown is as smooth as possible. Any dents or nicks in the wax will become obstructions in the mould and cause turbulence in the flowing metal.

4. Line the casting ring with a length or ring liner (it is easier to apply when damp). Check the crown margins and remove the wax pattern from the die. Weigh the wax pattern using a balance if you wish to determine the amount of alloy required.

5. Measure the length of the sprue against the casting ring, and adjust its height accordingly (aiming for the pattern to be 3–5 mm from the top of the casting ring).

6. Attach the sprue to the former using molten wax.

7. Place the casting ring onto the sprue former and check that the pattern is 3–5 mm from the top of the mould (place a tool over the top of the casting ring to help you judge this).

8. Also check that the wax pattern is central in the mould when viewed from above.

9. Spray the wax pattern with a surface tension reducer. Then gently dry with compressed air.

10. Metal casting investment is usually supplied in pre-weighed sachets.

11. Mix according to manufacturer's instructions, first-hand mixing in a vacuum pot to incorporate all the liquid.

12. Mechanically mix the investment under vacuum (the manufacturer's instructions will give – in seconds – the mixing, working and setting times).

13. Pour the material into the mould with the aid of vibration.

14. Care should be taken particularly as the investment reaches the wax pattern. Watch carefully to ensure no air is trapped.

15. Fill the mould to the top.

16. To ensure that no air has been trapped, you may pour the investment back into the mixing pot to ensure the wax pattern is coated evenly. Refill as before.

17. Refill as before, slightly overfilling the mould.

18. Fill the mould and leave to bench set according to the manufacturer's instructions, typically 30 minutes.

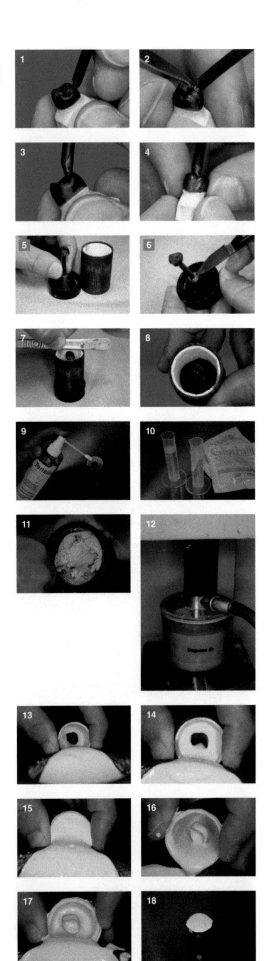

Investment material

For types I–IV gold, gypsum-bonded investments may be used. These have a fine particle size giving good surface detail, and are soft, which makes it easy to de-vest after casting.

Accurate castings are achieved as the TEC is matched closely to that of the gold alloys. The TEC needs to be matched so that the mould can be heated and expanded to compensate for the contraction of the metal after freezing.

Use of gypsum is limited to the lower melting temperature alloys as it breaks down at temperatures above 690°C, producing gases that affect the casting. The mould temperature needs to be high enough to prevent the molten metal from freezing as it enters the mould.

For bonding alloys and non-precious alloys, a 650°C mould temperature is not high enough. For example, nickel–chromium (Ni–Cr) alloy used often for metal-ceramic restorations has a melting temperature of approximately 1400°C. For this mould, a temperature of approximately 900°C is required so a phosphate-bonded investment material is required. These have the disadvantage that they are very hard and therefore difficult to de-vest; also the expansion is over a greater range and is therefore more difficult to match to the metal. They are mixed with colloidal silica to help control expansion.

Investing ▷ Casting and de-vesting ▷ Finishing the casting

4.6 Casting and de-vesting the pattern

Introduction

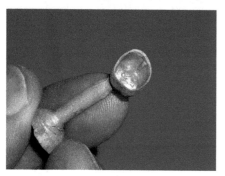

Figure 4.6.1

The mould is now heated and filled with molten metal. The mould is heated so that the molten metal does not freeze on entry, and also to provide expansion that will offset the contraction of the alloy upon cooling (this thermal expansion/contraction relationship is carefully worked out by the manufacturer of the investment and the alloy such that there is no overall dimensional change at the end of the process) (Figure 4.6.1).

Some investments require slow heating from room temperature (otherwise, they may fracture due to thermal shock). Other investments have been designed to withstand being put directly into a hot furnace, and do not require a long heating time. Regardless of the investment type, the mould must be given time to heat-soak, and so be of consistent temperature throughout.

There are many ways of heating the alloy and providing the force necessary to get the molten alloy into the mould. The following method uses electrical resistance heating, combined with centrifugal force for casting.

Work safety

Training is required in the use of any casting machine. Care should be taken in and around these pieces of equipment as very high temperatures are reached.

You will need:

- The set mould (from Section 4.5)
- Furnace
- Casting machine
- Heat source
- Alloy flux
- Plaster knife
- Furnace tongs
- Pickling acid solution
- Safety gloves and goggles

Basic procedure

1. Remove the rubber sprue former from the base of the casting ring, and trim any surplus investment from the top and sides.

2. Place the mould in the burnout furnace and adjust the temperature. Follow the manufacturer's instructions for recommended heating rate and temperatures as some recommend a staged increase (e.g. for Cristobalite the furnace temperature should be approximately 650°C).

3. The mould is allowed to heat-soak for approximately an hour to allow the mould to become hot all the way through.

4. Weigh out the metal alloy. Enough should be used to provide the force required to fill the pattern. Therefore, if using a metal of low density, a larger quantity will be required for the button. Use: Wax pattern weight × density of alloy (from manufacturer's data sheet) = weight of alloy for casting.

5. Once the mould has heat-soaked, start to heat the alloy in the crucible of the casting machine.

6. Observe the alloy melting (use tinted safety goggles). Once the alloy has lost form, take the mould from the furnace.

7. Place the mould on the casting arm of the casting machine (with the cone form facing the crucible). Align the crucible and mould. Close any safety shield and start the casting machine.

8. Once cast, retrieve the mould from the casting machine using tongs and put aside to cool.

9. Check that the mould has been filled (the 'button' of alloy should be complete).

10. If the mould appears to have not been completely filled, this is often due to an incorrectly aligned crucible causing a mis-cast. A partially filled mould may result in porous alloy or feathering to the thin edges of the casting due to a lack of casting force.

11. Once cooled, the casting is de-vested. Using a plaster knife, loosen the investment around the button.

12. For soft investment materials you should be able to easily push the casting from the casting ring using a plaster knife.

13. Break off the bulk of the investment material from the metal casting. It is advisable to keep the casting wet at this stage to reduce the dust created.

14. For hard investment materials, use a small hammer to repeatedly hit the button and break the refractory material.

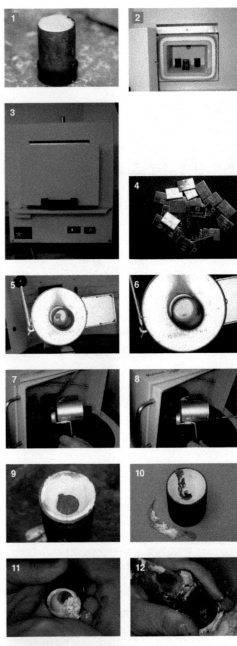
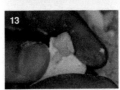
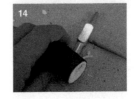

Continued over

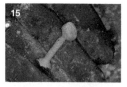

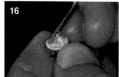

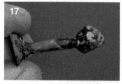

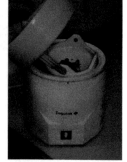

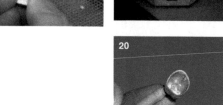

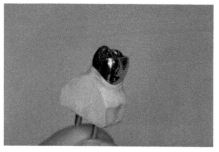

15. The completed casting will have a fine layer of surface oxide and debris.

16. Remove any remaining investment using a small brush or tool in water. Care should be taken to avoid damage to the casting, particularly at the margins.

17. The oxide remaining on the surface can now be removed.

18. For gold alloys, remove surface oxides by immersing into acid (pickling).

19. For non-precious metals, remove the investment by shot-blasting with 50 μm aluminium oxide. (For more on finishing bonding alloys, see Section 4.8.)

20. The casting is now ready for trimming and finishing.

Hints and tips

There are several different methods of heating the alloy for casting and also for applying the casting force.

- Casting forces: Centrifugal, air pressure and vacuum.
- Heat sources: Natural gas or propane mixed with either air or oxygen, acetylene mixed with oxygen, electrical resistance, electrical induction.

Investing ▷ Casting and de-vesting ▷ Finishing the casting

4.7 Finishing the casting

Introduction

The restoration is now ready for the final stages of production. The objective is to have a highly polished surface to the restoration, which is not only aesthetically pleasing but also prevents plaque and food adhesion and irritation of the tongue and soft tissues (Figure 4.7.1).

Figure 4.7.1

Work safety

Dust extraction and eye protection should be used when trimming and polishing alloys.

You will need:

- The de-vested casting (from Section 4.6)
- Micromotor
- Cut-off disc and mandrel
- Abrasive wheels and stones
- Rubber polishing wheels and points
- Bristle brush
- Cotton mops
- Rosehead metal bur
- Polishing compound
- Steam cleaner
- Acetone
- Articulating paper

Basic procedure

1. Gently try to seat the casting on the die. Do not use force. Remove the casting and inspect the fitting surface.

2. Areas preventing seating should be removed using an abrasive stone or small bur. These areas should be visible as the die spacer will lightly mark the fitting surface of the casting. Do not proceed until the restoration is fully seated on the die.

3. Using a carborundum cut-off disc, cut off the sprue as close to the restoration as possible, without compromising the shape of the crown.

4. Trim the excess alloy from the sprued area to restore the contour of the mesio-palatal cusp using an abrasive wheel.

5. Using articulating paper, check and adjust each contact point with its adjacent tooth. When checking the mesial contact remove the distal abutment tooth. This prevents the distal tooth from interfering with the seating of the crown. Similarly, remove the mesial abutment tooth when checking the distal contact.

6. Lightly adjust the contacts using a fine abrasive stone and repeat until the crown can be seated.

7. Finally, check both contacts simultaneously.

8. Using a fine abrasive stone, smooth the outer surface of the restoration to a consistent finish.

9. When using abrasives, care should be taken near the margin where the material is thin.

10. The surface should be of an even surface texture and free of porosity, before progressing to a finer abrasive. This applies to the finishing of all gold restorations.

11. To smooth the surface use an abrasive rubber wheel on the external surfaces. To avoid creating 'hollows' in the surface, use the wheel at about 10 000 rpm, making small circular movements.

12. An abrasive rubber point or cone at low speed may be used to smooth the occlusal area. A small rosehead metal bur may be used to carefully define the occlusal detail.

13. Use a bristle brush and suitable polishing paste to achieve the final polish. First apply the polish to a slow speed brush.

14. Running the brush slowly, apply to the restoration surface. The surface will initially become dull (as it becomes covered in the waxy polish). Make small circular movements with the brush covering the entire surface of the restoration until no scratches remain. Work on one small area at a time, in a logical sequence. You may need to apply more polish to the brush.

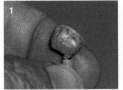
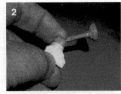
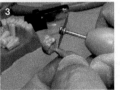
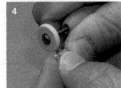
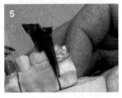
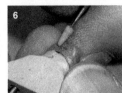
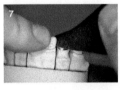
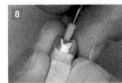
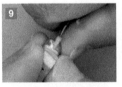
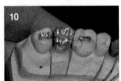
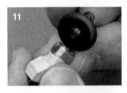
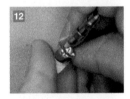
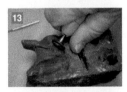
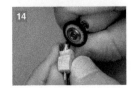

Continued over

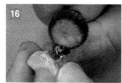
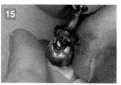
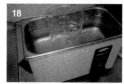
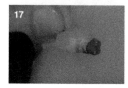
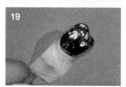

15. Smaller brushes are available to allow access to the occlusal detail.

16. Use a cotton mop and finishing compound (jewellers' rouge) to achieve a glossy surface. Again, the surface will first become dull before brightening. A clean cotton mop may be used to apply the final buff.

17. Clean the die using a steam cleaner.

18. To finish, the restoration may also be steam cleaned, or placed for 5 minutes in a solvent (such as acetone) in an ultrasonic cleaner.

19. Wash the restoration in water and fit back on the master model.

Extended information

Alloys for metal restorations

The main considerations for alloy types are cost, biocompatibility and corrosion resistance. Mechanical properties such as stiffness, strength, ductility and hardness all need to be suitable for the clinical situation in which the alloy is to be used. Consideration also needs to be given to the physical properties, such as melting temperature, density and thermal expansion for the technical procedure.

Generally when formulating such an alloy, the compromise is between the stiffness, which is a result of the elastic modulus and the design of the structure, and ductility, which is advantageous when burnishing. If making a supporting structure consideration also needs to be given to the resistance to permanent deformation, which requires high yield stress.

There are basically three groups of alloys used for metal restorations: gold alloys, palladium alloys, and non-noble metals (non-precious) such as cobalt–chromium (Co–Cr) or Ni–Cr.

Gold alloys

Gold alloys can be categorised into high, medium or low gold content.

High gold alloys (>75% noble metal content, Au, Ag, Pt, Pd) are sub-classified as types I–IV based on hardness: I soft; II medium, increase in Cu content; III hard; and IV extra hard.

Carats or fineness is not commonly used in dentistry to classify the amount of Au content. However, for information, carats are 24ths and fineness is in 1000ths. Therefore, 18 carat = 750 fineness = 75% Au. High gold dental alloys range from 21.4 to 14.4 carat (900–600 fineness).

Continued over

Alloying elements:

- Ag: Strengthens and counteracts the reddish tinge from the Cu.

- Cu: Increases strength; it is the most significant alloying element for strengthening as it gives rise to 'order hardening' (11% Cu is needed for this; maximum Cu is 16% as above this tarnishing occurs). Types III and IV can also be annealed to harden. Cu reduces the melting temperature.

- Pt: Increases the strength and melting temperature.

- Pd: Similar effects as Pt.

- Zn: Acts as a scavenger, preventing oxidation.

- Others include iridium, ruthenium and rhenium (<0.5%). These are usually added to act as nucleating sites to produce a fine grain size.

Use of high gold alloys:

- Type I: Inlays (low stress) – soft and easily deformed, low yield stress allows burnishing and high ductility means that they are unlikely to fracture.

- Type II: Most Inlays, although not in thin sections as deformation is possible.

- Type III: Inlays, onlays, full coverage crowns, short-span bridges, cast posts and cores. This is due to higher strength, although more difficult to burnish and a higher potential for localised fracture in the hardened state.

- Type IV: Cast posts and cores, long-span bridges and partial denture construction. (For partial dentures, clasps are adjusted in 'as cast' state, and then hardened.) These alloys have low elastic modulus and high yield strength; therefore, they have high flexibility and can spring out of undercuts without permanent deformation. They cannot be burnished.

Medium gold alloys

These range from 40% to 60% Au and have a greater content of Pd and Ag. Cu content is approximately 15%. Pd is used to stop the Ag tarnishing.

These are indicated for the same use as types III and IV high gold alloys. Ductility is generally lower and the high yield stress combines to make these alloys difficult to burnish and also results in a danger of fracturing. Suitable for long-span prostheses and implant-supported structures.

Low gold alloys

These range from 15% to 20% Au with 40–60% Ag and <40% Pd; therefore, these could be described as Ag–Pd alloys. In dentistry this name is reserved for alloys of <2% Au. These alloys tend to be white in appearance

Continued over

but some are coloured with indium. This creates a less homogeneous alloy that compromises the mechanical properties.

These alloys generally have poor properties and are therefore only recommended as a substitute for type III alloys. In addition, because they are white in appearance they are less popular and only used where coverage is possible, for example, post and core.

In Ag–Pd alloys, Pd again provides the resistance to tarnishing. These alloys generally require heat treatments to attain adequate properties. The properties do vary significantly but they are generally indicated for use as a substitute for type IV alloys. However, they are contraindicated for long spans because of their poor accuracy. This is due to the high melting temperature and the TEC being difficult to match with the phosphate-bonded investment materials required for such temperatures. They also tarnish and cannot be burnished.

Co–Cr alloys have now generally replaced type IV alloys for partial denture construction. Problems with the metal include very high casting temperatures, compromising accuracy. The increased hardness creates difficulties in polishing and the low ductility results in clasp fracture. The high modulus of elasticity though is advantageous in that the alloy is rigid in thin sections. It is also of low density and therefore extremely light – although low density can be disadvantageous with respect to casting.

4.8   Metal-ceramic restorations

Introduction

Metal-ceramic restorations were developed as a compromise between the superior aesthetics of all-ceramic restorations (porcelain jacket crown or PJC at the time) and the strength of all-metal restorations. Ceramics are inherently weak and must be supported in order to be clinically useful. The ceramic in metal-ceramic restorations gains it strength by being supported by the metal substructure.

A metal-ceramic restoration is composed of the following:

(1)   Metal substructure: Design and alloy composition are important.

(2)   Oxide layer: Critical in the bonding of the metal to the ceramic.

(3)   Opaque layer: Provides bond, obscures metal colour and initiates the shade.

(4)   Dentine ceramic: Major colour contributor and bulk of ceramic.

(5)   Enamel ceramic: Incisal and interproximal areas for translucency.

(6)   Glaze: Strengthening, hygiene and aesthetics.

Design of the metal substructure (framework or coping)

The metal substructure is typically produced using the lost wax process although other production methods used in conjunction with CAD are becoming popular. The design of the metal substructure is important as it provides the fit, support for the ceramic, emergence angle and occlusal and interproximal contacts.

The metal substructure must provide support for the ceramic, which should be limited to a maximum thickness of 1 mm. Ceramic in greater thickness is susceptible to fracture. The ideal method for creating a substructure that will provide support for the ceramic is to start with a fully contoured restoration in wax and cut this back by 1 mm for the ceramic. Then the wax restoration will then be invested and cast into metal.

In practice most substructures are produced by dipping the die in wax, producing a thin even layer, and adding wax to areas where the technician considers support is required. At worst, the wax is left as a thin layer and the ceramic built to the full contour. This increases the risk of failure of the restoration due to the unsupported ceramic cracking; however, it is done to save metal costs and production time.

When designing metal-ceramic restorations, consideration should be given to how much tooth substance has been removed and from where. Typically, the labial or buccal side of a preparation will have greater reduction and a shoulder margin to allow room for ceramic to be placed, whereas the palatal will have less reduction and a chamfered margin for a metal finish. The design of the junction between the metal surface and the ceramic surface is often the decision of the technician. Consideration must be given to the amount of tooth reduction, aesthetics and requirements for occlusal and proximal contacts.

Proximal contacts can be formed as part of the metal substructure or in the ceramic, but not at the junction between the two. This is because the junction can be abrasive and unhygienic. Likewise, the occlusal contact can be either metal or ceramic, but not at the junction of the two. Metal occlusal contacts have the advantage of being less wearing on the opposing dentition as they are less abrasive than ceramic. They are also easier to adjust and re-polish at the chairside.

The detail of the design needs to be considered to ensure that there is a suitable finishing edge for the ceramic and no sharp corners, which may cause stress concentrations.

Tooth preparation

- Reduction of at least 1.5 mm at the shoulder or anywhere else where ceramic is to be placed.

4.9 Producing a wax pattern for a metal bonded to ceramic framework

Ditching → Wax pattern production → Investing

A wax pattern is produced for the metal framework that will support the ceramic and replace the morphology of the tooth where required.

In this section, an example will illustrate a central incisor (Figure 4.9.1) and premolar (Figure 4.9.2). The principles illustrated can be applied to any other metal bonded to ceramic restoration.

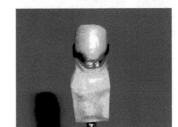

Figure 4.9.1

You will need:

- A ditched die on a sectional model
- The opposing model
- Die hardener
- Die spacer
- Wax knife, carver and Bunsen burner
- Tissue paper
- Separating medium
- Inlay wax
- Wax dipping pot (if available) or sheet casting wax

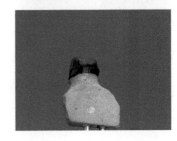

Figure 4.9.2

Basic procedure

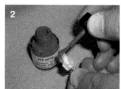
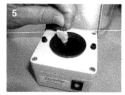
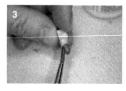
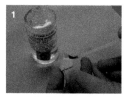
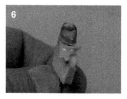
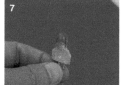
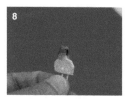
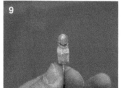
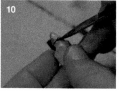
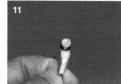

1. Cover the die with a thin coat of die hardener and remove excess using compressed air. There should be no residual material on the surface of the die.

2. Apply two coats of die spacer to allow room for the luting cement. This should finish 1 mm above the margin to ensure a tight marginal fit.

3. Once dry, apply separator to the die, adjacent and opposing teeth, using a brush. Remove the excess using compressed air or a tissue paper.

4. To form the initial wax layer of the framework, either the die can be dipped in molten wax or a sheet of casting wax (see steps 7 and 8) can be applied to the die.

5. Turn on the wax dipping pot and allow the wax to melt completely. Dip the die into the molten wax until the margins are submerged, remove and allow to solidify.

6. A drip always forms; this can be reduced by touching it on the rim of the pot, or alternatively, hold the die such that the drip will harden where extra wax is required (such as the tip of a cusp) – go to step 9.

7. If using sheet casting wax to form the initial wax layer, gently fold this around the preparation.

8. Join the free ends together using wax.

9. The soft dipping or sheet wax is replaced with a harder wax in the marginal area (this maintains the accuracy of the margin). Remove a 1 mm strip of wax above the margin from the initial layer using a knife or carver.

10. Fill the void with molten inlay wax (or suitable hard modelling wax).

11. Once the wax is cool, smooth the join using a carver (removing any excess wax that may have gone over the margin). At this stage, it is worth ensuring that the pattern can be removed and replaced on the die.

12. The ideal shape of the framework is best created by first building the restoration to full contour, and then removing 1 mm of wax from those areas where ceramic is to be placed. Alternatively, the framework is thickened in areas where more support is required.

13. For an anterior restoration go to step 14, and for a posterior restoration go to step 21.

Continued over

Anterior restoration

14. Add wax to extend the coping to form contact points with the adjacent teeth and continue to form the shape.

15. The contour should contact and harmonise with the adjacent teeth and contact occlusally with the opposing tooth.

16. Create a recording of this shape to assist the cut back, using silicone putty.

17. Using a warm knife, make 1 mm deep incisions into the wax in the area to be reduced.

18. The silicone recording may be sliced to create an index (or matrix).

19. Hold the index against the model to check the amount of reduction. There should be 1 mm of space for the ceramic. Note that the contact point with the lateral has been left in place and will eventually become a metal contact.

20. The palatal aspect also remains at full contour, which will result in a metal palatal surface (final restoration shown for clarity).

Posterior restoration

21. Add wax to extend the framework to form contact points with the adjacent teeth and continue to form the shape.

22. Add wax incrementally to build support for cusp tips using the opposing model as a guide.

23. Add wax to the lingual/palatal aspects of the restoration and continue to build to full contour. The restoration should harmonise with the adjacent teeth.

24. Ensure that the functional cusps are in contact with the opposing teeth. When correct, create a recording of this shape to assist the cut back using silicone putty.

25. The silicone recording may be sliced to create an index (or matrix).

26. Using a warm knife, make 1 mm deep incisions into the wax in the area to be reduced.

27. Hold the index against the model to check the amount of reduction. There should be 1 mm of space for the ceramic (here, to the distal surface of the buccal cusp).

28. The junction between the metal and ceramic should be contoured such that a hygienic finish is produced and rounded to prevent stress concentrations.

Continued over

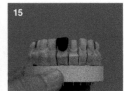
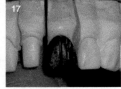
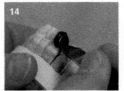
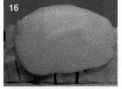
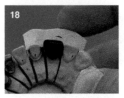
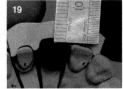
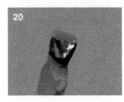
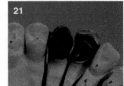
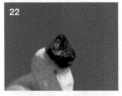
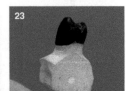
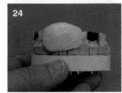
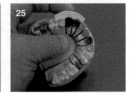
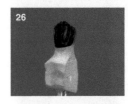
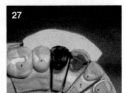
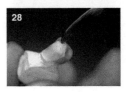

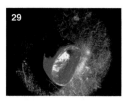

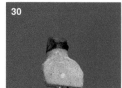

29. Once finished, remove the wax pattern from the die.

30. Prior to investing check the marginal fit, emergence profile, adjacent and occlusal contacts and ceramic finishing junction.

Note: Patterns for metal substructures are often produced as an even thickness of wax, with additions to support the ceramic (rather than building to full contour and cutting back 1 mm). This technique is quick and easy, but does compromise the strength of the finished restoration, as the ceramic is not adequately supported.

Wax pattern production ⟩ Investing ⟩ Casting

4.10 Investing the wax pattern

Introduction

A mould of the wax pattern is now made from a refractory material.
Follow the instructions in **Section** 4.5, but note these considerations:

- Bonding alloys have a high melting temperature (to withstand the high temperatures during sintering of the ceramic). Therefore, a refractory investment material which can withstand these higher temperatures, such as phosphate-bonded material, must be used.

- Depending on the alloy being used, the sprue diameter might need to be increased. Check the manufacturer's recommendations.

Investing ⟩ Casting ⟩ De-vesting and finishing the casting

4.11 Casting the pattern

Introduction

Follow the instructions in **Section** 4.6, but note these considerations:

- The mould must be heated to a significantly higher temperature (typically 900–950°C). Check the manufacturer's recommendations.

- The heat source for the casting machine needs to be able to reach temperatures exceeding 1200°C.

Extended information

Bonding alloys for metal-ceramics

Alloys for metal-ceramic restorations (bonding alloys) are specifically designed for the purpose and differ from type I–IV alloys for the following reasons:

Continued over

- They must produce a metal oxide that is essential for forming bond with the ceramic.

- The TEC should match that of the ceramic – it has been suggested that it should be slightly higher than that of the ceramic, which would allow the alloy to shrink slightly more on cooling and result in the ceramic being kept under compression.

- The melting temperature must be higher than the sintering temperature of the ceramic; otherwise, the alloy will start to deform or melt as the ceramic is fired.

- They must have a high elastic modulus and yield strength (be stiff), and therefore not flex under load; otherwise, ceramics can crack or 'ping' off.

- They must not contain any elements that may discolour ceramics.

It is not possible to use types I–IV gold alloys because of the following:

- Their TEC is not compatible with the ceramics.

- They have a low melting temperature and therefore would deform at sintering temperatures.

- Will not bond to ceramics, as they contain no base metal to form oxide.

- They are not stiff enough.

High gold alloys

These alloys are very successful for metal bonded to ceramic restorations as they are strong and create a good bond with the ceramic. The melting temperature is raised by the addition of platinum and palladium. Their main disadvantage is that the melting temperature is low; therefore, they are susceptible to creep at high temperatures. They also have a lower elastic modulus and must be used at a minimum substructure thickness of 0.5 mm. This can give rise to problems with aesthetics in some situations. There is no copper in these alloys as this reduces the melting temperature, and also reacts with the ceramic causing greening.

Gold palladium alloys

These were introduced to lower costs. They are comparable with high gold in terms of castability, accuracy, fit and corrosion resistance; however, the TEC can be more sensitive and the alloy is incompatible with some ceramic systems.

High palladium alloys

These alloys may contain copper, but this does not affect the functional properties of the alloy. Sag resistance can be poor; therefore, they must not be used for long spans. This alloy is gaining popularity.

Continued over

Palladium–silver alloys

These have the most favourable elastic modulus of all precious metal alloys. They have low flexibility and reduced tendency to sag, but are less forgiving in terms of castability and fit. Silver can cause discolouration and therefore require careful alloy–ceramic combinations.

Nickel–chromium alloys

These alloys are very stiff, with elastic modulus 2.5 times that of high gold; therefore, coping thickness can be reduced to 0.3 mm and long-span bridges are less flexible. They are unlikely to sag because of high melting temperatures. Casting is difficult and accuracy compromised due to very high melting temperatures (approximately 1450°C). The metal–ceramic bond is also less reliable. This alloy is used for minimal preparation bridges, as the surface can be etched to make it suitable for bonding.

Casting › De-vesting and finishing the casting › Ceramic application

4.12　De-vesting and surface preparation

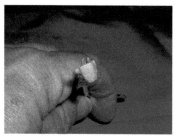

Figure 4.12.1

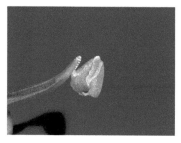

Figure 4.12.2

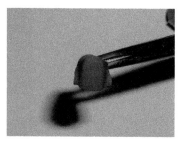

Figure 4.12.3

Introduction

The bond between metals and ceramics can be quite temperamental and it relies heavily on the surface treatments of the metal. This requires care when trimming the pattern. Ensure that suitable abrasives to create the correct surface roughness are used, either non-contaminated tungsten carbide burs or ceramic-bonded abrasives.

Follow the instructions in **Section** 4.6, but note these considerations:

- Trim the surface in one direction to avoid trapping debris (Figure 4.12.1). The burs used should be 'ceramic bonded'.

- The surface should have no sharp edges to act as crack initiation points. Shot-blast the outer surface to give suitable surface irregularities for micro-mechanical retention and clean in an ultrasonic cleaner (Figure 4.12.2).

- Some manufacturers suggest that the metal substructure should then be put through a heating cycle to de-gas and oxidise the metal surface (Figure 4.12.3). See Extended information below.

Extended information

Oxidation: Noble metal alloys with only small amounts of base metal do not oxidise readily. (The oxide layer is necessary for bonding). Therefore, the alloys are first put through a heat cycle to create an oxide layer on the metal. Base metals do not require this as they oxidise readily; the oxide layer would be too thick and weak.

Continued over

Degassing: This is the same procedure but done for a different reason. The idea is to burn off any organic debris on the surface and allow any trapped gas in the surface layer to diffuse out.

Bonding mechanisms of metal to ceramic

Bonding is not fully understood but is known to rely on the following:

- van der Waals forces: Secondary bonds – minor attraction between opposite charges. These rely on close proximity; therefore, good wetting of the surface is necessary. The oxide is required to attain good wetting.

- Mechanical retention: This is gained from microscopic surface irregularities. Again, good wetting is essential for the ceramic to flow into the details. Shot-blasting creates the correct surface. However, again, this is only a minor contributor to the overall bond strength.

- Compression bonding: This is achieved by matching the TEC of the metal and ceramic such that the ceramic contracts slightly more than the metal on cooling. This results in the ceramic being able to cling to the metal substructure. Conversely, it is also advocated that the metal should shrink more than the ceramic in order to pull the ceramic into constant compression.

- Chemical bonding: This is the single most significant mechanism and is a bond utilising the metal oxide. The surface oxides dissolve into the opaque layer of ceramic that allows atomic contact with the metal surface. The oxide layer effectively increases wetting, allowing direct chemical bonding so that the ceramic and metal share electrons. Both covalent and ionic bonds form. This mechanism requires only a molecular layer of oxide; if excessive oxide is formed the result is a sandwich effect and the ceramic will not come into contact with the metal.

4.13 Ceramic application and build-up

Casting > De-vesting and finishing the casting > Ceramic application

Introduction

Ceramic is applied and fired onto the metal substructure using the sintering process. The ceramic is supplied as a finely ground powder that is mixed with a fluid to form a wet mix (Figure 4.13.1). This is then added to the substructure and shaped using a brush or spatula. The excess moisture is drawn from the build-up using tissue, and the ceramic particles condensed such that they are tightly packed together.

Once the desired shape is achieved, the ceramic build-up is fired at approximately 900–1000°C, allowing the particles to sinter together (Figure 4.13.2).

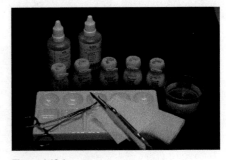

Figure 4.13.1

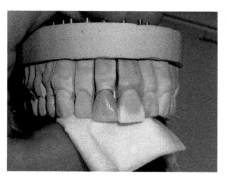

Figure 4.13.2

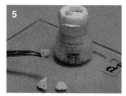

Figure 4.13.3

Ceramic application: wash opaque layer

Applying the wash opaque; this is a very thin layer that creates the bond between metal and ceramic (Figure 4.13.3).

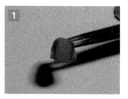
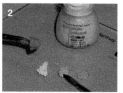
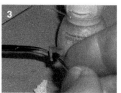
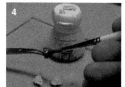
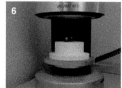

Basic procedure

1. Load the tweezers with the substructure, holding by the collar.

2. Mix a small quantity of the wash opaque ceramic to a thin paste in a palette, or on a glass slab using a glass mixing rod.

3. Wet the substructure surface with a small amount of modelling fluid.

4. Wet your brush and pull it backwards across tissue whilst twisting. This should form a neat point to the bristles. Lift a small amount of the paste using the brush and place it onto the labial surface.

5. Drag the ceramic paste out to the margins of the restoration and the metal–ceramic junction.

6. Place the framework on a firing stand and fire according to the manufacturer's instructions.

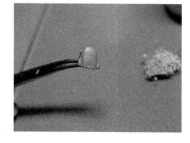

Figure 4.13.4

Ceramic application: opaque layer

The opaque layer is a thicker layer of material that ensures the metal does not show through the ceramic and also establishes the restoration's shade (Figure 4.13.4).

Basic procedure

1. Using the correct shade, mix the opaque ceramic in the palate with the appropriate modelling fluid to a thick mix that is almost capable of holding its shape.

2. Holding the substructure in the tweezers, shape your brush to a point and pick up a small amount of material. Place this on the incisal edge of the restoration and using your brush, drag it such that it forms a line of material from the incisal edge to the margin.

3. Blot the moisture from the opaque ceramic strip by gently holding the tissue against the side of the ceramic. You will see that the watery, shiny surface disappears and gradually becomes matte.

4. Vibrate the metal framework by gently dragging the serrations on the shank of your spatula over the tweezers once or twice. You will see that the surface becomes shiny again as the ceramic particles settle to the metal framework and the moisture comes to the surface. Blot the moisture with tissue.

5. Take your brush and place another strip of ceramic next to the first such that they touch.

6. Vibrate once or twice gently using the spatula, as before. The two should join as the moisture rises to the surface.

7. Blot as before. Any irregularities that occur may be smoothed by using your brush. Draw this between your fingers to make a small fan shape; this can be used to delicately smooth the surface.

8. Repeat this process all the way around the framework until completely covered.

9. Place the framework on a firing stand and fire according to the manufacturer's instructions. When fired, if any grey shadows are visible through the opaque layer, add some more ceramic and repeat the firing process.

    The same procedure is used for posterior restorations.

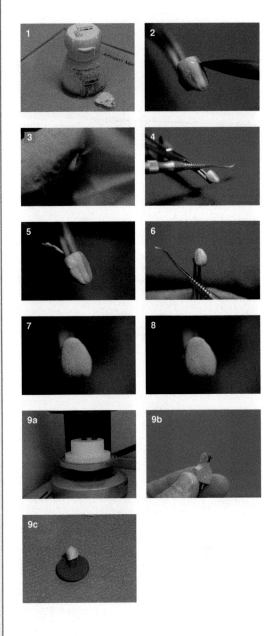

Ceramic build-up

The bulk of the ceramic may now be placed. Base dentine and enamel shades are used to build to full contour (Figure 4.13.5).

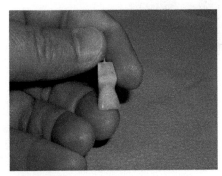

Figure 4.13.5

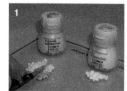

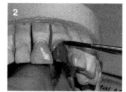

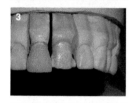

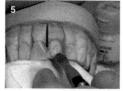

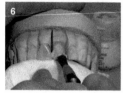

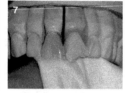

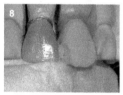

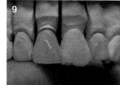

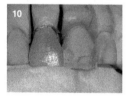

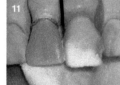

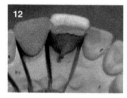

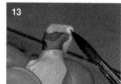

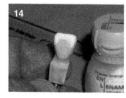

Basic procedure

For an anterior restoration

1. Mix the dentine material to a thick mix as before.

2. Coat the adjacent and opposing teeth with separator.

3. Place the framework on the die, ensuring that it is fully seated.

4. Hold a tissue against the incisal edge of the restoration. Then, lift a small amount of ceramic on a pointed brush or ceramic spatula.

5. Place the ceramic against the substructure taking care to avoid trapping air; condense using the tissue to blot excess moisture.

6. Build up the ceramic incrementally and condense as you go. Try not to let the ceramic dry out completely as it will become difficult to carve.

7. Start building one surface of the restoration to full contour. The ceramic will shrink on firing so over-build the restoration by approximately 10%.

8. Avoid filling the interproximal areas with ceramic, as this will cause difficulty in removing the ceramic.

9. A fan-shaped brush is again useful for moving or smoothing the ceramic.

10. Cut back the incisal edge using the spatula to create room for the translucent enamel ceramic. This should be done according to the clinician's prescription.

11. Mix and place the enamel ceramic into the void created and smooth the surface. Remember that the ceramic must be moist to allow the dentine and enamel powders to blend, and that on firing the material will shrink by 10%.

12. Check the palatal aspect to ensure the ceramic meets the metal junction and the shape harmonises with the adjacent tooth.

13. Remove the die from the model to allow access to the interproximal areas and contact points. Add ceramic to these areas to create the full contour of the crown.

14. The restoration is now ready for firing. Owing to the ceramic being over-built to compensate for firing shrinkage, it cannot be fitted back onto the model.

15. Fire the ceramic using the appropriate firing cycle.

Continued over

For a posterior restoration

1. Follow the basic principle as for the anterior restoration. Coat the adjacent and opposing teeth with separator and apply a layer of base dentine ceramic to the framework.

2. Working logically, build up the base dentine ceramic to full contour, using the opposing model as a guide if necessary.

3. Cut back the dentine layer, and replace it with enamel ceramic. Smooth using a brush.

4. Complete the occlusal surface, overbuilding by 10% to account for firing shrinkage. Remove the die from the model and add ceramic to the proximal contact points.

5. Fire the ceramic using the appropriate firing cycle.

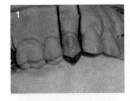
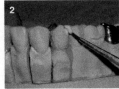
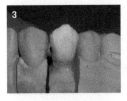
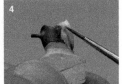
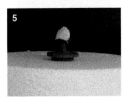

Ceramic additions, trimming and finishing

It is extremely rare that the restoration is of the correct size and shape after the first firing. The next stage is to trim the restoration to correct the contact points so that it fits back on the model. Fine adjustments to the shape of the crown are made by grinding with burs, or deficient areas can be added to with an additional firing (Figure 4.13.6).

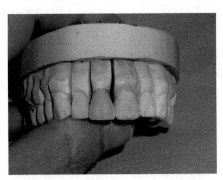

Figure 4.13.6

Basic procedure

For an anterior restoration

1. Gently attempt to seat the restoration on the die. The contact points should be tight, preventing the seating of the restoration.

2. Mark the contact points by placing articulating paper in between the restoration and adjacent tooth, or alternatively lightly rub the contact area of the adjacent tooth on the model with pencil lead and replace the crown. The pencil lead will mark the tight contact.

3. Lightly reduce the restoration where it has been marked using a diamond or ceramic abrasive bur.

4. The best technique is to check one contact point at a time, by removing the adjacent teeth from the model.

5. Repeat until the restoration seats fully without excessive force.

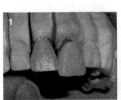
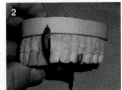
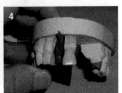
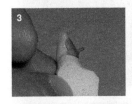
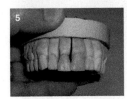

Continued over

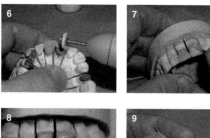

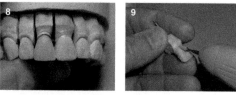

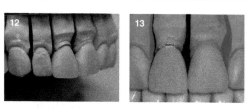

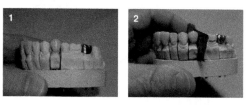

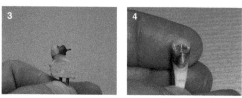

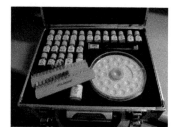

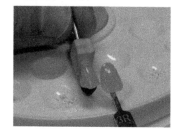

6. Shape each surface of the restoration in turn. First check the incisal edge and reduce or reshape as required to match the adjacent tooth.

7. Looking from the incisal edge, trim the labial surface to match the contour of the adjacent tooth.

8. Trim the mesial and distal aspects of the restoration to create the correct shape when viewed from the labial aspect.

9. The cervical area should be contoured to blend into the margin.

10. Check the palatal aspect, trim to match the adjacent teeth and to allow the opposing teeth to contact.

11. Clean the restoration using water and ceramic to any deficient areas. The ceramic will not shrink greatly during this second firing; therefore, place only the required amount of material.

12. Fire the ceramic and adjust as necessary.

13. Remove the glossy surface from the ceramic prior to glazing.

For a posterior restoration

1. Gently attempt to seat the restoration on the die. The contact points should be tight, preventing the seating of the restoration.

2. Check the contact points as described for the anterior restoration.

3. The ceramic is adjusted using the diamond or ceramic-bonded burs.

4. The occlusal surface should be checked to ensure that there is a smooth transition between the metal and ceramic.

5. Ceramic may be added using the same method as described for the anterior restoration.

Figure 4.13.7

Ceramic glazing and staining

Once the desired shape is achieved the ceramic is glazed and stained where necessary. The correct stain powder (Figure 4.13.7) is chosen using the shade guide and is applied at the same stage as the glaze (Figure 4.13.8).

This outermost layer forms a hygienic finish for the ceramic, allows the surface to be matched to the adjacent teeth and improves the strength of the restoration.

Figure 4.13.8

Glazing powders

(1) Mix the desired staining powders with glazing liquid and apply to the ceramic surface using a fine brush (Figure 4.13.9).

(2) Fire in the furnace using the appropriate cycle. The surface will have a high gloss finish (Figure 4.13.10).

Self-glaze

(1) Mix the desired staining powders with glazing liquid and apply to the ceramic surface using a fine brush.

(2) Fire in the furnace using the appropriate cycle. The surface should have a light glaze.

Finishing

(1) Polish all metal surfaces (except the fit surface) using fine abrasives and rubber wheels (Figure 4.13.11).

(2) Clean the restoration by placing in acetone in the ultrasonic cleaner for 5 minutes (Figure 4.13.12).

(3) Steam clean the models (Figure 4.13.13).

(4) Seat the restoration on the model.

(5) The restoration, model and opposing model should be returned to the clinic.

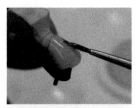
Figure 4.13.9

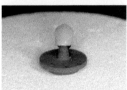
Figure 4.13.10

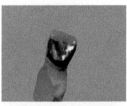
Figure 4.13.11

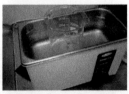
Figure 4.13.12

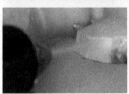
Figure 4.13.13

Extended information

Providing a ceramic margin or shoulder

When the restoration margin is likely to be visible, a ceramic margin is indicated. The metal framework is designed such that it finishes at the internal angle of the preparation shoulder. The opaque layers are applied as normal. Producing ceramic in this region requires an additional stage to be completed prior to the main build-up.

1. Liberally apply separator to the die, seat the framework and apply the margin ceramic in a thick consistency to the restoration. Fill the entire void to create a smooth transition between the margin and the opaque layer.

2. Carefully remove the framework and fire the ceramic.

3. A second application is often required to produce a satisfactory finish.

The metal substructure may also be designed to provide support for a partial denture or to carry a precision attachment (intra or extra-coronal).

Continued over

Hints and tips

- Use a pencil to outline areas for trimming.
- When trimming, use a fast speed but low pressure to avoid heating the ceramic and wearing the diamond.
- Copy the surface detail from the adjacent tooth.
- Wipe the ceramic surface with water to see how the restoration will appear when glazed.

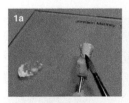

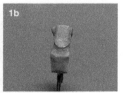

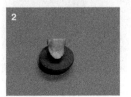

The ceramic is fired in a programmable vacuum furnace. This allows accurate temperature control for specific times and the vacuum ensures minimal porosities in the fired ceramic. When firing a bulk of ceramic it is necessary to allow adequate drying time; failure to do this will result in the trapped moisture vaporising quickly and causing the ceramic to blow off. Once fired, the core material will be opaque and relatively tough. The aesthetic veneering ceramics can now be applied.

For the simplest restorations a minimum of two veneering ceramics are used. These are the base dentine and the enamel shade. The base dentine provides the shade for the prescribed restoration and the enamel is used to provide translucency at the incisal edge or cusp tips.

For advanced shade matching, opacious dentines, translucent dentines, opal ceramics and a range of effect dentines are available that together can be used to build complex restorations. The limiting factor with modern ceramics is the capability of the dentist to prescribe accurately and the technician to produce the prescription.

A typical firing cycle would be: Dry at 600°C for 5 minutes; raise to 930°C over 7 minutes under vacuum; and hold at 920°C without vacuum for 1 minutes. Cool to 600°C over 2 minutes. The ceramic is cooled slowly; failure to do this would result in the outside cooling far quicker than the inside. As a result, the outside would contract more inside and fracture would occur.

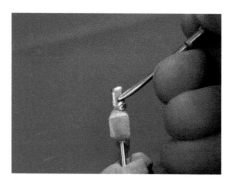

Figure 4.14.1

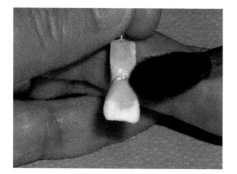

Figure 4.14.2

Figure 4.14.3

4.14   Ceramic restorations

Introduction

Until recently, three types of all-ceramic restoration were in use: PJC, resin-bonded crown (also known as dentine-bonded crown) and high-strength ceramic substructure crowns. Of these, the PJC has been superseded by the newer high-strength and/or bondable materials.

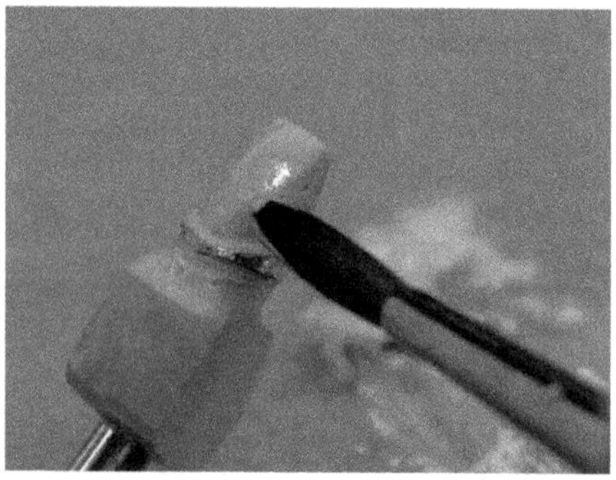

Porcelain jacket crown

The PJC may be considered the first all-ceramic restoration. They are produced by adapting a platinum foil around a die on to which the ceramic is built (Figure 4.14.1). The foil supports the ceramic as it is removed from the die and placed in the furnace for firing.

The core of the restoration is built from an aluminous porcelain (high content of alumina). This is significantly stronger than feldspathic porcelain (veneering ceramic) and provides the necessary strength. The disadvantage is that the core is very opaque and therefore requires ample veneering ceramic to mask it (Figure 4.14.2).

Onto the fired aluminous porcelain core, feldspathic veneering ceramics, which are supplied as powders, are applied using a brush (Figure 4.14.3). The aesthetics that can be achieved are impressive; however, the strength of the final restoration is limited by the aluminous core material, which is substituted in modern high-strength ceramic restorations.

PJCs have relatively good aesthetics, are hygienic, have a thermal conductivity similar to that of teeth and are relatively cheap (Figure 4.14.4).

Once the firing stages of production are complete, the foil is removed prior to fitting the crown (Figure 4.14.5).

PJCs can be produced on a refractory die (duplicated from the original). This avoids the foiling procedure as the ceramic is fired on the model. Once complete the refractory is removed using a shot-blaster. The material to produce PJCs is slowly being phased out by some manufacturers due to the popularity of other types of all-ceramic restorations. However, the use of a platinum foil to support ceramics is still in use today in the production of porcelain laminate veneers or resin-bonded crowns.

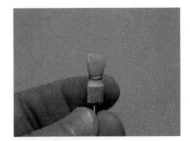

Figure 4.14.4

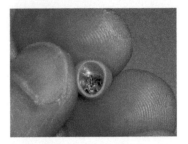

Figure 4.14.5

Resin-bonded restorations

Resin-bonded restorations have no high-strength core material. They rely on using a veneering ceramic that has the ability to be acid etched and bonded to the tooth. Strength is gained from the tooth structure rather than a tough core. These are called dentine-bonded crowns, resin-bonded crowns or 360° veneers. Veneers are produced using the same method and materials.

They are generally produced from sintering ceramics on a refractory die although other production methods are possible. The main advantage of this type of restoration is that there is no opaque core material resulting in a restoration that is aesthetically superior and requires less tooth reduction (Figure 4.14.6).

Alternative processing routes are available for these restorations. The first is CAD–CAM (Figure 4.14.7).

Restorations may be processed from an industrially produced ceramic block using CAD–CAM techniques (Figure 4.14.8).

These materials are stronger and quicker to produce than sintered ceramics. The ceramic block is of a single colour relying on surface staining for colour matching or on the technician to cut back and add enamel ceramics. Colour-graduated blocks are available, although limited in application.

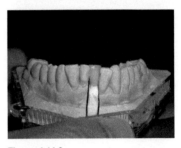

Figure 4.14.6

Lithium disilicate materials (e.g. Ivoclar Emax)

These materials are significantly stronger (PJC approximately 80 MPa, feldspathic ceramic approximately 150 MPa, lithium disilicate approximately 500 MPa and zirconia approximately 1000 MPa). The material may also be etched to enable resin bonding, further increasing the strength of the cemented final structure.

The range of available shades and translucencies enables this material to be used as a monolithic restoration, that is, the restoration is produced from one shade, which may be characterised and glazed. Alternatively, the material may be used as a substructure on to which ceramic may be sintered in the usual way. The versatility, strength and aesthetic properties of this material have led to it becoming a popular choice.

The choice of processing route also caters for the preferred method of the dental technician as it may be processed via hot-pressing using the lost wax process, or via CAD–CAM.

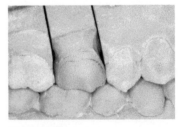

Figure 4.14.7

High-strength ceramic substructure restorations

This type of restoration gains its strength from high-strength substructures that support the veneering ceramic.

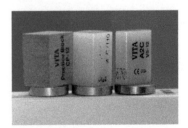

Figure 4.14.8

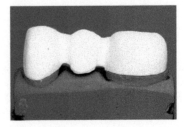

Figure 4.14.9

There are several different materials available that differ in translucency and strength, the majority of which are processed via CAD–CAM, although slip casting of some materials is possible.

Zirconia: (approximately 1000 MPa flexural strength) This material is produced via CAD–CAM and is milled approximately 20% larger than the desired dimensions. On sintering at high temperature (approximately 1400–1500°C) the material shrinks to the correct size. Each batch of material is labelled with the shrinkage factor that is programmed into the machining software. It is available in different translucencies and can be stained to the correct shade prior to sintering. The very high strength of these materials enables their use for the construction of long-span bridges.

Alumina: (approximately 500 MPa flexural strength). This material can be processed in a similar way to the zirconia materials, although it is not as strong, limiting its application to single units and anterior bridges.

Glass-infiltrated materials: There are a range of these materials based on alumina which are processed via CAD–CAM or can be slip cast. Vita In-ceram produce versions named spinell, alumina and zirconia, which increase in opacity and strength in this order. The differences give rise to their clinical indications for use. Spinel (400 MPa): single anterior units, Alumina (500 MPa): Single units and anterior bridges, Zirconia (600 MPa): Single units and bridges.

Tooth preparation: all-ceramic high-strength framework:

- Shoulder reduction of between 1.0 and 1.5 mm is required depending on the ceramic (see the manufacturer's instructions).

4.15   Producing a high-strength ceramic substructure

Introduction

High-strength ceramic substructures are increasingly produced using CAD–CAM production methods (either in the dental laboratory or in a dedicated milling facility). Another method is slip casting, although this is becoming less popular as CAD–CAM becomes increasingly affordable and convenient. Irrespective of the production methods, the substructure produced is high-strength alumina, or more commonly, zirconia. Each is veneered using feldspathic ceramics.

It is outside the scope of this book to give detailed instructions for each system, but an overview of the methods is given below.

Slip casting

Slip casting was one of the early methods for producing high-strength ceramic substructures. The framework is first produced from an alumina slurry (the slip) on a refractory die, and lightly sintered. The porous material is subsequently infiltrated with a low-viscosity glass, which gives it its high strength and translucency. The substructure is veneered using feldspathic ceramics.

CAD–CAM systems

Numerous systems are now available for the dental technician to allow for CAD–CAM of high-strength substructures. These systems feature either digital or touch scanning equipment to create a three-dimensional digital representation of the die in a computer by scanning the working model. The digital restoration is then milled in the dental laboratory using a bench-top milling unit. Depending on the system, a selection of materials may be used, ranging from composite and plastics to bondable ceramics to high-strength core materials. See Section 4.25 for more detail.

External processing centres

Similar to the laboratory-based CAD–CAM systems, specialist software is again used to design the substructure, but is instead sent electronically to a remote milling centre. This has the advantage that expensive milling equipment is not required in the dental laboratory.

4.16 Veneering a high-strength ceramic substructure

Introduction

The high-strength substructure is veneered to create the full contour of the restoration, in the correct shade and surface finish to match the adjacent teeth.

A high-strength substructure is veneered using feldspathic ceramics in the same way as for a metal bonded to ceramic restoration (Section 4.13) but with the following considerations:

- The thermal expansion coefficient (TEC) of the veneering ceramic must match that of the substructure (see manufacturer's instructions). Whilst bonding alloys have a TEC of approximately 13 ppm, zirconia has a TEC of 9 ppm and alumina a TEC of 7 ppm.

- The opaque step is omitted, as the substructure is tooth coloured.

4.17 Producing a resin-bonded crown on a refractory die

Ditching → Refractory model production → Ceramic application

Introduction

Resin-bonded restorations are produced from ceramics that may be acid etched and bonded to the tooth. The materials used are not particularly strong, but once bonded, they are supported by the tooth structure.

Sintering is the most popular method of production. The complication with resin-bonded restorations is that there is no ceramic substructure that may be used to transport the ceramic powders to the furnace. To overcome this problem, a refractory die is produced to support the ceramic during firing. Alternatively, a platinum foil may be adapted over the die and used to support the unfired ceramic. In both cases the support is removed once the restoration is complete and the restoration fitted to the original model.

CAD–CAM may also be used to machine a resin-bonded restoration from a block of ceramic (see Sections 4.27 and 4.28 for more information). There are several methods of producing a refractory die.

- Pour a second model from the impression in a refractory material. Although quick, the disadvantage of this method is that it does not produce a sectional model on which to build the ceramics. It may also be difficult to remove the relatively weak refractory material from the impression.

- Produce the sectional model as normal, remove the die and make a mould using a laboratory silicone. This method is more time consuming but has the advantage that the refractory die can be used in the sectional model. The silicone used is very flexible and allows easy removal of the refractory die.

- If using a sectional model in a tray system, produce a sectional model as normal, and then take an impression of the sectioned model using a flexible silicone. Take the impression of the model, remove the die to be duplicated and cut a hole in the bottom of the tray. Replace the impression and pour refractory material through the hole in the tray. Once set, remove the impression and delicately take out the refractory die.

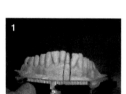
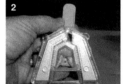
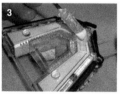
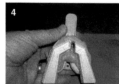
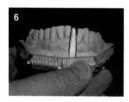
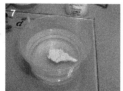
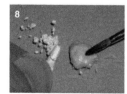
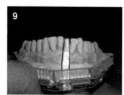

Basic procedure

1. Take an impression of the master model using a low-viscosity silicone impression material.

2. Remove the impression and die from the model and using a bur, cut a hole in the tray base where the die locates.

3. Apply separator to the adjacent sections of the model, reassemble and pour a die using refractory material.

4. Once set, remove the tray base and model sections from the impression.

5. The refractory die should be fired according to the manufacturer's instructions prior to commencing the ceramic build. The margin may be highlighted at this stage.

6. Fit the sections into the tray and base.

7. Soak the die in water to prevent the ceramic drying out during ceramic application.

8. Apply a thin wash of ceramic to the die and fire to seal the refractory material and create the inner surface of the restoration.

9. Ensure that the fired ceramic has flowed over the surface of the refractory material.

Continued over

10. Build the ceramic to the full contour as described in Section 4.13.

11. When firing the ceramic, ensure that the restoration does not contact the muffle of the furnace. Also be aware that the temperature may need to be increased to heat-soak the large volume of material.

12. The ceramic should be shaped using diamond or ceramic-bonded stones.

13. The ceramic is glazed and stained as required.

14. Once the ceramic work is finished the restoration can be removed from the refractory die.

15. Use a diamond disc to section the refractory material close to the restoration.

16. Use a narrow bur to remove the bulk of material from the inner fitting surface of the restoration.

17. Use a shot-blaster with 50 μm glass bead at low pressure (2 bar) to remove any remaining material. Be careful to ensure that the surface finish is protected during this procedure. Wax may be used to cover the surface.

18. Coat the die with occlusal indicator spray, or as here with lipstick, and seat the crown gently.

19. Remove and gently trim any areas preventing full seating of the crown.

20. Clean the restoration in an ultrasonic cleaner in acetone, and steam clean the die.

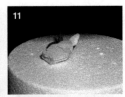
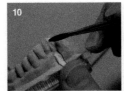
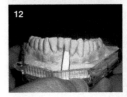
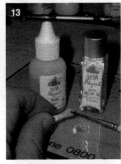
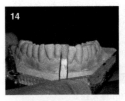
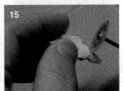
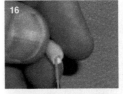
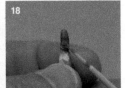
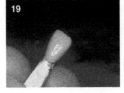
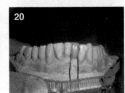
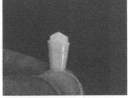
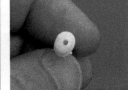

4.18 Post crowns

Ditching   Post production   Impression

Introduction

Post crowns are used to restore teeth that have broken down to such an extent that the crown of the tooth is almost non-existent (shown in Figure 4.18.1 on an artificial tooth for clarity).

The tooth is endodontically treated; the pulp chamber of the tooth is cleaned out and enlarged (Figure 4.18.2) to allow for a metal restoration to be placed within.

The restoration is often produced as two parts, the 'post and core', and a separate crown is produced to fit this. It is possible to produce a one-piece post crown; however, this is uncommon.

Core design

In the post crown technique the core is designed and produced by the technician. The contour of the core should be designed to follow the preparation design for that of a natural tooth. The core should be two-thirds the length of the original

Figure 4.18.1   **Figure 4.18.2**

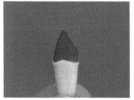

Figure 4.18.3

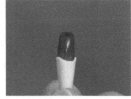

Figure 4.18.4

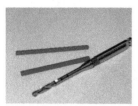

Figure 4.18.5

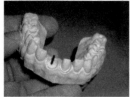

Figure 4.18.6

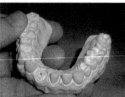

Figure 4.18.7

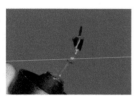

Figure 4.18.8

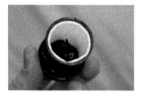

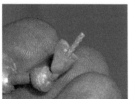

Figure 4.18.10

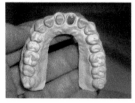

Figure 4.18.9

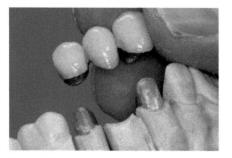

Figure 4.18.11

crown with all angles gently rounded providing adequate retention and resistance for the overlying restoration (shown in Figure 4.18.3 in red).

An even shoulder, normally 1 mm wide, should be formed around the root face. The proximal surfaces should be almost parallel in the vertical plane and palatally inclined in the horizontal plane. The cingulum area should be near parallel to the labial surface. The incisal third of the labial surface should have a lingual curve (Figure 4.18.4).

Overview of producing an indirect post and core in the laboratory

(1) Pre-formed (e.g. ParaPost): This system comprises of matching reamer and plastic posts: one smooth, one serrated (these are available in a range of sizes) (Figure 4.18.5).

(2) The tooth is reamed out and the matching smooth post fitted. An impression is taken and the post withdrawn from the tooth as part of the impression. The model is then cast in the laboratory and the post transferred to the model (Figure 4.18.6).

(3) The smooth sides of the post allow it to be removed from the model (Figure 4.18.7).

(4) The serrated post is inserted into the model and the core produced in wax around it (Figure 4.18.8).

(5) The post and core incorporating serrated 'burnout' post is invested and the plastic post is burnt out along with the wax (Figure 4.18.9).

(6) The detail of the serration is transferred to the gold casting (Figure 4.18.10).

(7) The sprue is removed and the casting trimmed to the original contour (Figure 4.18.11).

(8) This is returned to the clinic and cemented in place (where the serrated edges of the post aid retention). A further impression is taken, and a crown produced to fit.

Direct post and cores

The technician plays no part in the provision of direct post and cores. The clinician fits reams to the tooth, and fits one of the commercially available posts. A core is built around this post using appropriate restorative material.

Ditching > Bridge design > Cast metal fixed-fixed restoration production

4.19 Bridges

Introduction

A dental bridge is a restoration designed to replace one or more missing teeth and comprises at least one abutment-supported retainer and one pontic (Figure 4.19.1).
Bridge component/terminology (Figure 4.19.2):

- Abutment: a tooth that supports a bridge (1)

- Pontic: an artificial tooth that spans a gap between abutments (from pont, French for bridge) (2)

Figure 4.19.1

- Retainer: the restoration, typically a crown, cemented to the abutment tooth (3)
- Connector: the term used for the junction between two units of a bridge (4)
- Pier: an intermediary abutment between pontics
- Unit: each component of the bridge, retainer or pontic is referred to as a unit.

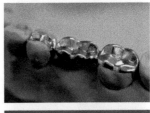

Figure 4.19.2

Types of bridge

There are four types of conventional bridge (i.e. a bridge that is cemented into place, rather than resin bonded):

(1) Fixed–fixed: This has two retainers supported by abutments, one at each end, with at least one pontic in between (Figure 4.19.3). Modifications may be made to add further abutments (e.g. four-unit bridge).

(2) Fixed–moveable or semi-fixed: This has two retainers and a pontic; however, it contains a joint that allows vertical movement of a retainer (Figure 4.19.4).

(3) Cantilever: A cantilever bridge has one retainer supporting a pontic from one side only (Figure 4.19.5). Modification may be made to add more abutments.

(4) Spring cantilever: This bridge has a retainer distant to the pontic, connected by a flexible arm (Figure 4.19.6).

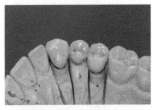

Figure 4.19.3

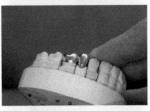

Figure 4.19.4

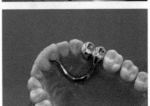

Figure 4.19.5

Pontic design

The design of the pontic should be a clinical decision. Consideration is given to:

- Aesthetics
- Occlusion with the opposing tooth
- Contact with the gingival tissues
- Prevention of food impaction
- Oral hygiene maintenance by the patient.

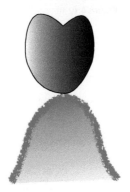

Figure 4.19.6

There are four recognised pontic designs:

- Bullet or dome shaped (Figure 4.19.7)
- Saddle shaped (Figure 4.19.8)
- Ridge-lap (Figure 4.19.9)
- Self-cleansing (wash-through, sanitary, hygienic) (Figure 4.19.10).

When producing a pontic you should ensure the following:

- The occlusal surface is narrowed bucco-lingually to reduce the occlusal forces placed upon it.
- Embrasures are designed to allow cleaning.
- The pontic should make light contact with the mucosa.

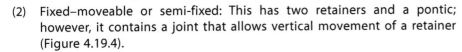

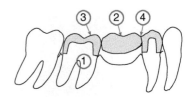

Figure 4.19.7

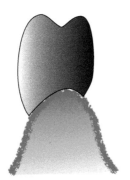

Figure 4.19.8

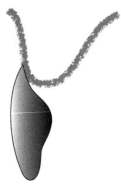

Figure 4.19.9

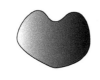

Figure 4.19.10

- If a metal–ceramic pontic is being used, that the junction between the ceramic and metal should be clear of the soft tissues. Similarly, the junction should not form the contact with adjacent and opposing teeth. The metal substructure should be designed to support for the ceramic.

Connectors for all metal bridges

Connectors join the component parts of a bridge together. Connectors should be designed as large as possible to provide sufficient strength to resist occlusal forces applied to the pontic. The dimensions are often limited due to aesthetics or contact with the soft tissues. The ideal dimensions of connectors are given in Table 4.19.1.

Table 4.19.1

Location	Height (mm)	Width (mm)	Indicated for:
Anterior	2.0	2.0	Small single pontic bridges
Anterior	2.5	2.5	Larger multiple pontic bridges
Posterior	>2.5	>2.5	Single, or multiple pontic bridges

Connectors for metal-ceramic bridges

The retainers of the restoration are produced as for single-unit substructures. Difficulties often arise when designing the connectors for metal-ceramic bridges. The design is a compromise between strength and aesthetics. For optimum aesthetics, a bulk of ceramic should be present to mask the underlying metal structure. However, for optimum strength the metal connector should be as large as possible, therefore limiting the thickness of the ceramic veneer.

Problems may arise when providing enough room for the ceramic in order to hide the metal substructure at the join between abutments. A concave connector edge is provided on the connector to allow for improved aesthetics.

Occasionally, for example, in a short clinical crown, this may significantly reduce the area of the connector, thereby weakening the structure. In this situation the connector may be extended into the occlusal surface of the abutment.

Connectors for all-ceramic bridges

All-ceramic bridges are produced in one piece with the connectors designed into the framework. As with the cast metal fixed–fixed bridges, this is only possible where the preparation of multiple fixed units are parallel to each other.

Fixed–fixed bridge

This type of bridge is relatively simple to construct, and is considered robust and to have maximum retention. This makes fixed–fixed bridges the most practical for long spans. They are produced and cemented as a single piece with a single path of insertion and therefore require the preparations to be parallel. This may be difficult to achieve without substantial tooth reduction in poorly aligned teeth. The rigid connection between the abutments acts to splint the teeth together; therefore, the entire occlusal surface of the abutment must be covered by the restoration. If a minor connector was used, de-cementation may occur.

The joints between the units are usually cast as part of the framework, although in some circumstances it may be necessary to solder or laser weld the alloy frameworks together. All-ceramic restorations are always designed as one piece.

Fixed–fixed bridges may be extended to comprise multiple abutments with one or more acting as a pier abutment or multiple pontics; however, all are rigidly connected.

Material selection

The criteria for selection are the same as those for metal, metal-ceramic or all-ceramic single-unit restorations with the complication of ensuring the connector and pontic are strong enough (see Table 4.19.1). The design depends on the health and position of the abutment teeth. The materials allowing minimal destruction of tooth tissue are generally indicated with compromises made for aesthetic requirements, allergy or cost.

Preparation requirements

Feather or chamfer margins used with cast high gold alloys provide the most reliable marginal integrity due to the materials being malleable and ductile.

Porcelain fused to metal or high-strength ceramic restorations require shoulder preparations to allow adequate thickness of ceramic. Consequently, they are more destructive to the tooth.

4.20   Producing a cast metal fixed–fixed restoration

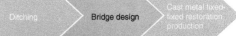

Ditching > Bridge design > Cast metal fixed–fixed restoration production

Introduction

A fixed–fixed restoration may be produced entirely from a metal alloy, or alternatively a metal–ceramic design may be used for improved aesthetics. For all-ceramic bridges, CAD–CAM techniques are employed (Figure 4.20.1).

For all-metal bridges the basic procedure follows that of single-unit restorations (see Section 4.4). The bridge can either be cast whole or in individual units and soldered together (used for long spans when there is concern about the accuracy of the casting process).

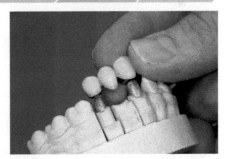

Figure 4.20.1

You will need:

- Wax knife
- LeCron carver
- Bunsen burner
- Inlay wax
- Sectioned, ditched, hardened and spaced model

Work safety

Be careful with hot waxes, and observe all safety warnings when casting metal.

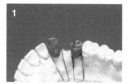
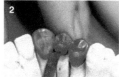
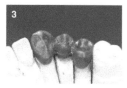
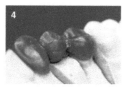
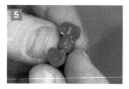
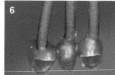
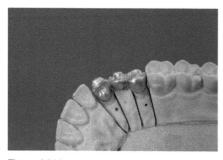

Basic procedure

1. Produce the wax pattern for the retainers as described for metal restorations.

2. Create a pontic to bridge the gap between the abutments.

3. With the retainers seated fully, attach each of the wax components to one another. Care should be taken to avoid damage to the existing patterns and to maintain the interproximal margin.

4. Ensure the connector is large enough.

5. Remove the wax pattern and ensure each wax connector is complete and free from voids.

6. Sprue and invest ensuring the size and number of sprues are adequate. Normally a sprue should run to each unit, either individually or through a feeder bar.

Bridge design ▷ Soldered metal fixed- fixed restoration production ▷ Soldering ▷

4.21 Producing a soldered metal fixed–fixed restoration

Introduction

Long or complex bridges may require the wax pattern to be split for the purpose of casting, as the accuracy of a casting reduces with an increase in length (small distortions are amplified across the length of the pattern) (Figure 4.21.1). This technique may also be employed where individual units are produced from different alloys.

Figure 4.21.1

You will need:

- Wax knife
- Bunsen burner
- Modelling wax
- Strengthening wire, rod or similar
- Refractory material
- Solder with melting temperature lower than that of the alloys used
- Soldering flux
- Burnout furnace
- Furnace tongues
- Gas torch to heat the alloy and solder (low temperature gold solders use gas and compressed air, high temperature gold solders use a oxygen–propane mix, and for nickel chrome alloys use a fierce oxygen–propane mix)

Work safety

Be careful with hot waxes, and observe all safety warnings when casting metal.

Basic procedure

1. Assemble the components on the model and ensure correct seating. A gap of 0.5 mm should be present between the surfaces to be soldered.

2. Secure the components to each other using wax or a self-curing acrylic resin. Use a strengthener (such as a discarded bur shank) to add rigidity if necessary.

3. Lift the bridge from the dies and check that there has been no displacement of components or fracture of the securing material.

4. Mix the refractory material as recommended by the manufacturer and pour against the fitting surface of each retainer unit until completely filled.

5. Place a small mound of refractory onto a flexible flat surface and place the restoration on so the occlusal surfaces are uppermost and the margins are covered with investment.

6. On setting, trim to reduce overall size to a minimum, as less bulk will make the assembly easier to heat evenly.

7. With a scalpel create a smooth 'V' shaped channel leading towards each connector in order to allow access with the flame and solder.

   Soldering is described in Section 4.22.

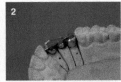
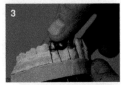
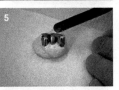
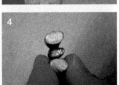
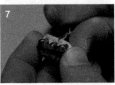
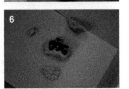
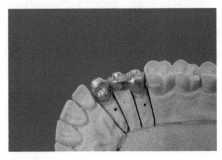

Extended information

If the components are to be located intra-orally, a plaster impression of the occlusal surfaces should be used providing a location key, should the parts separate in transit.

Hints and tips

Soldering

- Avoid over-heating. This causes melting or deformation of thin sections and porosity or excessive flow of the solder.
- Under-heating solder causes a 'dry' (weak) joint.

Metal-ceramic restorations

- Ensure any ceramic surface is relieved with paraffin wax.
- In addition to pouring the refractory material into each up-turned retainer and inverting onto a mound, allow the refractory to cover any relieved ceramic.

4.22 Soldering

Introduction

Soldering may be required to extend contact points on metal restorations, to join multi-unit bridges or to repair a broken or sectioned bridge (Figure 4.22.1).

Figure 4.22.1

You will need:

- Wax knife
- Bunsen
- Modelling wax
- Strengthening wire, rod or similar
- Refractory material
- Solder with melting temperature lower than that of the alloys used
- Soldering flux
- Burnout furnace
- Furnace tongues
- Pickling acid
- Gas torch to heat the alloy and solder: Low temperature gold solders use gas and compressed air, high temperature gold solders use a oxygen–propane mix, and for nickel chrome alloys use a fierce oxygen–propane mix.

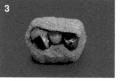
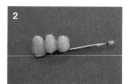
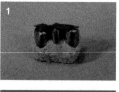
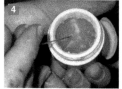
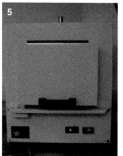
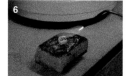
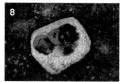
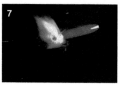
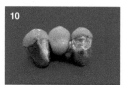
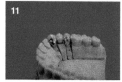

Basic procedure

Preparing metal components ready for soldering (all-metal restorations or *pre-ceramic* soldering)

Preparing components for *post-ceramic* soldering

1. To avoid contact between the ceramic and investment material (which cause degradation of the ceramic), the ceramic surfaces should be covered in a thin layer of modelling wax.

2. Invest as in stages 5–7 above.

Soldering

3. Boil away any wax residue to minimise carbon formation during soldering.

4. If necessary (see Extended information) apply a flux to the surfaces being soldered.

5. Place in a burnout furnace and raise the temperature gradually, close to the solder's melting temperature.

6. Remove from furnace and place on a heat-resistant surface and heat the assembly with a gas torch until red hot.

7. Touch the surfaces to be soldered with solder whilst maintaining the temperature using the flame.

8. As the molten solder is drawn through the gap remove the heat. The solder should look shiny and bright. Repeat until sufficient solder has been applied.

9. Gently remove the refractory investment before pickling in acid solution.

10. Trim any excess solder and reshape the connector using grinding stones.

11. Return the restoration to the model and check the marginal fit and occlusal contacts. Adjust and polish.

Flux (meaning 'flow') allows the solder to flow over the metal surfaces to be connected by preventing the formation of oxides on the metal surface during heating. Oxides prevent the solder from wetting and coming into contact with the metal surface.

Anti-flux is used as an aid for controlling the flow of solder. It is applied to areas where solder is not required or may cause damage. Common anti-fluxes are graphite (pencil lead) or proprietary anti-flux pastes.

Solders come in a variety of types for use with different metal alloys. The alloy datasheet provided by the manufacturer should recommend an appropriate solder. In general, the solder's melting temperature is significantly lower than that of the alloy being soldered. Modern solders are also available with flux included into the core of the stick to make melting and application easier.

Soldering may be classified as 'Furnace' or 'Flame' techniques. Flame soldering is described above. To carry out furnace soldering, the flux, solder and anti-flux are applied to the cold assembly. This is heated in a porcelain furnace to the liquidus temperature of the solder. Owing to the bulk of refractory, the furnace temperature may need to be increased by as much as 50°C to allow sufficient heat-soak for the solder to flow. The main advantage of furnace soldering is that the temperature can be controlled accurately, which is particularly useful when soldering restorations involving ceramic.

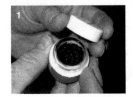

4.23 Minimal preparation bridges

Introduction

Minimum preparation designs offer a conservative method of tooth replacement with tooth preparation primarily restricted to the lingual surfaces of abutment teeth. They differ from conventional bridges in that they are resin bonded to the tooth structure as opposed to being cemented in the conventional manner. The high bond strength achieved enables the design of the bridge to rely on the resin bond for retention rather than the mechanical design for conventional bridges. For minimal preparation bridges it is only necessary to remove sufficient tooth substance to accommodate the retainer within the occlusion (Figure 4.23.1).

The retainer or wing must

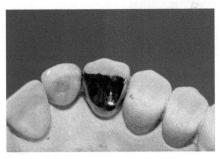

Figure 4.23.1

- fit closely to the prepared surface;

- be rigid on completion;

- cover adequate surface area to provide retention through bonding.

These bridges may be categorised as fixed–fixed, cantilever and spring cantilever (rigid cantilever bar). They are used in the case of single anterior tooth loss where a natural diastema occurs.

They are also categorised by the type of bonding that they use (see Extended information in Section 4.24).

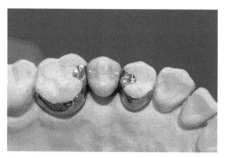

Figure 4.24.1

4.24 Producing a minimal preparation bridge (Maryland technique)

This type of retention can only be achieved with Ni–Cr alloys. This alloy develops retentive features when etched with acid or electrolytically (Figure 4.24.1).

Work safety

Be careful with hot waxes, and observe all safety warnings when casting metal.

You will need:

- Section refractory model
- Inlay wax
- Wax knife
- LeCron carver
- Bunsen burner
- Magnification

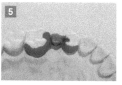
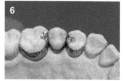
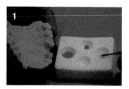
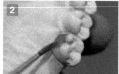
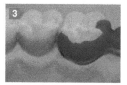
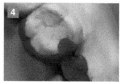
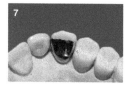

Basic procedure

1. Use monomer and polymer applied with a brush; first apply the separator onto the abutment teeth.

2. Using low-expansion polymethylmethacrylate (PMMA), construct the retainer wings (apply powder directly to the model and fix with monomer).

3. Follow the outline of the prepared surface on the abutment tooth, ensuring a wing thickness of 0.5 mm.

4. For posterior bridges, create an occlusal stop to distribute the load applied to the pontic. Ensure that this does not interfere with the opposing teeth.

5. Adjust the shape of the wings and create the pontic using inlay wax.

6. Sprue, invest, cast and apply the veneering ceramics (use the same technique as for metal bonded to ceramic crowns – see Sections 4.10–4.12).

7. Figure 7 is an example of a cantilever design.

Extended information

The Maryland-type minimal preparation bridge is the most commonly used of the type. The main types of minimal preparation bridge are classified by the type of bonding mechanism they use. These include the following:

- Macro-mechanical: This has large countersunk perforations in the retainer through which composite flows to provide retention. Rochette developed this technique for periodontal splinting. It is less retentive over time than other bonding mechanisms.

Continued over

- Medium-mechanical: (Virginia Salt Mesh, Crystal Bond). All methods involve retentive features cast as part of the metal framework; for example, the Virginia Salt method involves salt being applied to an adhesive on the die and the wax pattern being built on this. The pattern is then removed and the salt dissolved out. The pattern is then cast. The size of retentive features is intermediate between macro and micro systems and the retainer wing is thicker and requires greater occlusal clearance than wings manufactured for etchable non-precious alloys. It can be used with metals that do not etch, and hence metals without nickel components (important due to nickel sensitivity and allergy in some patients).

- Micro-mechanical: developed at the University of Maryland, giving rise to the popular name of Maryland bridge. Micro-mechanical retention is produced by electrolytic or acid etching the fitting surface of the retainer. These retainers do not have any non-retentive areas as do the medium-mechanical retentive systems. They also allow a thinner film thickness of cement and a retainer wing thickness of 0.3 mm.

- Electrolytic etching using chairside equipment is also possible and some reports suggest these techniques have been superseded by sand-blasting alone.

- Sand-blasting the retention wing's fitting surface using 50 μm aluminium oxide powder at around 2 bar pressure: This increases surface area and roughness, and the application of a silane coupling agent increases bond strength.

- Chemically adhesive (e.g. Panavia Ex): Chemically retentive resins are available. They adhere chemically to recently shot-blasted metal surfaces and are retained to the tooth by conventional acid etching of the enamel.

Micro-mechanical and chemically adhesive systems have been shown to be the most retentive. The disadvantage of micro-mechanical systems is that if they are tried in the mouth they must be refinished (etched) prior to bonding. This is because the delicate surface becomes contaminated.

Macro-mechanical systems overcome this problem but are less retentive; this is mainly due to the use of conventional composites to cement them rather than a specifically designed one as for other minimal prep bridges. The composite that comes through the holes is also susceptible to degradation. The main advantage, however, is that they can be removed easily by drilling the cement from the perforations. For this reason, they are still used when modifications are likely, that is, as an intermediate whilst tissue heals or when the prognosis of the abutment is poor.

Medium-mechanical systems were developed in an attempt to overcome the problems of the systems above; however, they are less retentive than micro-mechanical systems and have thicker metal retainers and cement film. One advantage is that medium-mechanical systems can be made from any metal whereas micro-mechanical relies on etchable metals.

Other less commonly used methods have been developed – tin plating or silica-coated – and each method produces a surface layer to which a silane coupling agent is applied to enable resin bonding to occur.

Continued over

4.25 Digital dentistry

Introduction

As with other technologies in their infancy, formats are not standard between manufacturers, in this case giving rise to 'Closed' or 'Open' systems. This results in software only being compatible with particular hardware and difficulties in exchanging data between different systems. This problem appears to be resolving slowly with more devices and software being marketed as open source.

Laboratory scanners

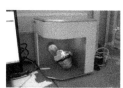

Figure 4.25.1

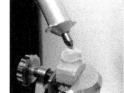

Figure 4.25.2

There are many scanners available for the dental laboratory that can be used to scan impressions, models, individual dies, bite registrations and waxed up restorations.

The majority of scanners are optical meaning that they use reflected light to acquire the data from the surface being scanned. Touch scanners are also available, which use a probe to record the surface (Figure 4.25.1).

Increasingly, scanners are stand alone units that may be used to gather data that can be exported to any software package for manipulation. The optical scanner shown scans a full model in 1–2 minutes allows additional scans to be added if necessary and has the functions of scanning all of the items mentioned previously (Figure 4.25.2).

Intra-oral scanners

Intra-oral scanners allow the capture of data directly from the mouth therefore having the advantage that an impression is not required. Restorations may be produced directly from the digital data and milled either at the chairside (the Chairside Economical Restoration of Esthetic Ceramics (CEREC) system being the most widespread) or in the laboratory. The range of restorations that can be produced via this route is limited to single units and restorations produced from one material, for example, composite or monolithic ceramic.

In order to produce restorations with a ceramic or composite veneer, a model would be required to enable the technician to fabricate the veneering layer in the usual way. Similarly, producing a restoration of more than one unit is unlikely to be advocated without a model, due to the need to check the accuracy of fit and contacts.

The production of models from data acquired digitally is an established route to avoid the need for an impression. Here, the digital data is used to 3D print a plastic model for use in production of the restoration or simply for checking the digitally produced restoration.

Other data sources

MRI & CT: Increasingly, dental software packages help the easy import of data from other sources such as magnetic resonance imaging (MRI) and computerised tomography (CT) scanning to enable more detailed planning of procedures involving the tissues underlying and surrounding the teeth. This data is particularly useful when planning implant procedures.

CAD software packages

Software packages are becoming very similar in the functions that are available and are continually updating to include new features. The applications for designing crowns, bridges and other indirect restorations are very sophisticated and the user interface is intuitive to the dental technician. Applications for removable partial dentures (RPDs), splints and full dentures are generally less well developed but are likely to catch up in the near future.

Details to consider when looking at these software packages:

- Is the software open to import from any scanner and export to any production route?

- What functions do you need and which are available as add on modules if you decide to change later?

- What is the annual cost for the licence, support and updates for the software?

- What training is supplied and what level of ongoing support is available and who provides this? As an end user you may find that another technician can provide the best support.

- What other software will you need to run your scanner or a milling unit?

A list of CAD packages is provided below; there are many more but these should give a good overview. Note that some of the dental companies used the same CAD package from a third party. The reader is referred to the companies' websites to see the latest offerings.

- 3Shape (3Shape)

- Exocad (Fraunhofer)

- Dental Wings

- Cerec (Sirona)

- Procera (Nobel Biocare)

- Zirkonzahn

- Incise (Renishaw)

- MultiCAD (KaVo – Fraunhofer)

CAM may be considered as subtractive manufacturing where a blank of material is reduced via a computer-controlled milling process, or as additive manufacturing whereby the item being produced is built in layers from a reservoir of the material.

Each has its own merits; milling is well established with a lot of manufacturers supplying equipment, resulting in a competitive market and relatively cheap equipment. The range of materials processed in this method is extensive, although the waste material is substantial.

Additive manufacturing, including 3D printing of wax for patterns and plastics for models, is well established for prototyping in other industries and is becoming of significance in dentistry. Similarly, laser sintering of metals is commercially available. The main obstacles are the cost of equipment and the production time. Unlike milling, each material requires a different machine for production, resulting in this type of technology being sited in a specialist production house.

Some dental laboratories have established themselves as production houses, taking digital designs and producing the item via the most appropriate method, be it milling, printing or laser sintering. This negates the need for individual laboratories to acquire and maintain the manufacturing equipment.

Presented below is a summary of the different materials that may be processed:

Milling (Figure 4.25.3)

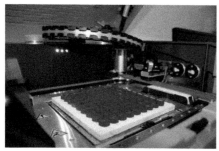

Figure 4.25.3

- Precious and non-precious metals: for indirect restorations and bars

- Wax: for patterns

- PMMA: for patterns and temporary restorations

- Pre-sintered zirconia: for substructures or full contour restorations

- Ceramics (feldspathic and lithium disilicate): for substructures or full contour restorations

- Glass-infiltrated ceramics

- Composites: for full contour restorations

- Hybrids: for full contour restorations

- Poly (aryl ether ether ketone) (PEEK): for implant-supported frameworks or RPD

- Poly (aryl ether ketone ketone) (PEKK): for substructures or full contour restorations

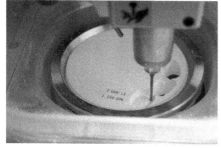

Figure 4.25.4

3D Printing (Figure 4.25.4)

- Wax: for patterns

- Photo-curing resin: for RPD patterns

- Plastics: for models

Selective Laser Melting (Figure 4.25.5)

- Precious and non-precious metals: for substructures, full contour restorations and RPD frameworks.

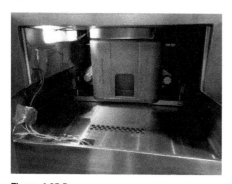

Figure 4.25.5

4.26 Using a laboratory-based CAD–CAM system

Each CAD–CAM system differs slightly; therefore, the procedure below outlines the basic steps (Figure 4.25.3). (Here a Medit Identica Blue scanner is being used with Exocad software before being milled using a Roland DWX-50).

Producing a Simple Substructure

Introduction

This simple production method creates a substructure of a given thickness uniformly over the surface of the die. The pattern may be edited manually using the design tools.

You will need:

- A sectional model produced in a scannable die stone (or powder spray)
- Millable material blank (e.g. zirconia, glass-infiltrated material)
- Glass infiltrating powder (if required)
- CAD–CAM scanner and milling system

Work safety

CAD–CAM systems have failsafe measures to prevent injury (which should not be tampered with). Dust and eye protection should be used when trimming die stone and the substructure material.

Basic procedure

1. Remove the die from the model. If a scannable die material has been used, this can be placed directly into the scanning holder. Normal die stone does not readily scan so will require a coating of reflective powder.

2. Place the die centrally in the rotational cup holder with the margin at the rim height. Fill around the die with the putty, staying 1 mm clear of the margin. Position the holder in the scanner with the mesial aspect of the die facing the front of the machine.

3. Load the software and create a new patient entry. Select the restoration to be produced and the tooth to be restored. Select 'Acquire preparation' and choose the rotational scan method.

4. Once the scan is complete, the software will render the scan into a three-dimensional image of the die.

5. Using the software, identify the margin of the preparation. When all the margin is marked, the software allows for any errors to be edited.

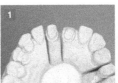
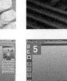
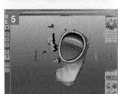

Continued over

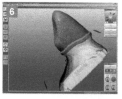

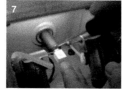

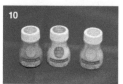

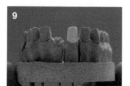

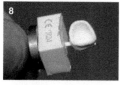

6. Select 'next' and the software will design your substructure (to the present parameters). You may adjust the wall thickness, occlusal thickness, or overall shape using the design tools.

7. When complete, select the 'Mill' option and load the appropriate material block into the milling machine.

8. The milling process is automated, and once complete the restoration can be retrieved (this takes 10–15 minutes).

9. At this stage, the substructure may be adjusted using a diamond bur. Typical adjustments are removing the sprue, alterations to the fit, and the emergence profile.

10. At this stage the material is weak, and will require further processing – either sintering or glass infiltration. Refer to the manufacturer's instructions for the material used.

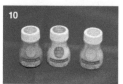

Figure 4.26.1

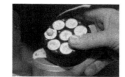

Figure 4.26.2

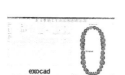

Figure 4.26.3

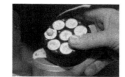

Figure 4.26.4

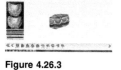

Figure 4.26.5

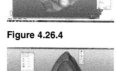

Figure 4.26.6

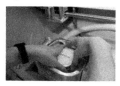

Figure 4.26.7

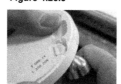

Figure 4.26.8

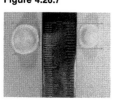

Figure 4.26.9

Procedure

(1) Create the work record in the software package detailing the type and position of the restoration (Figure 4.26.1).

(2) Scan the die by inserting it into the holder and working through the scanning wizard (Figures 4.26.2 and 4.26.3).

(3) Using the design package, work through the wizard to create a simple coping (Figures 4.26.4 and 4.26.5).

(4) Save the restoration design and export to the CAM software for milling (Figure 4.26.6).

(5) Set the material blank into the milling unit and work through the CAM software to create the tool path (Figure 4.26.7).

(6) Once the milling unit has completed, the item will need to be removed from the blank, adjusted and processed accordingly. Shown here is a zirconia coping which requires sintering (Figures 4.26.8 and 4.26.9).

4.27 Producing a posterior single-unit substructure or restoration using a reduction technique

Introduction

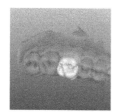

Figure 4.27.1

This technique allows the restoration to be designed to full contour, and accurately reduced by 1 mm where veneering ceramic is to be applied (Figure 4.27.1). In order to create a full contour restoration, the opposing dentition must also be captured by the design software.

The method for capturing and designing is similar to that of the single-unit substructure in Section 4.26, but with the addition of the opposing model to the data captured.

Basic procedure

1. Using scannable bite registration material, create an occlusal registration between the working and opposing models in the intercuspal position. The registration should cover the die and adjacent teeth.

2. Once set, remove the registration from the models and trim it so that only half the occlusal surface of each adjacent tooth is covered.

3. The occlusal surface is captured using multiple scans. These are aligned using a grooved locating surface.

4. In this case, two scans are required to form the complete image of the die and adjacent teeth.

5. Two further images are taken to record the bite registration (here called the antagonist).

6. The restoration is designed to full contour, taking into account the opposing and adjacent teeth.

7. The reduction function allows the entire surface to be cut back by 1 mm. At this stage, the restoration can be milled.

8. Alternatively, highlight the area that you wish to reduce, for example, a buccal facing, and selectively reduce this area. This restoration would be made from a bondable ceramic, or produced in metal by laser sintering or the lost wax process using a millable wax substitute.

9. For a complete cut back, the milled substructure should be processed and veneered as for a high-strength ceramic substructure crown (see Section 4.14).

10. For a partial cut back, select the ceramic system that matches the thermal expansion of the substructure material and build and characterise the restoration.

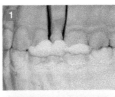
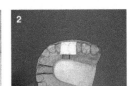
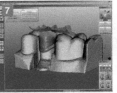
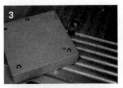
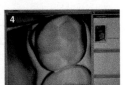
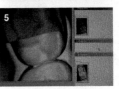
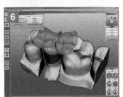
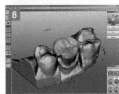
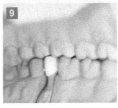
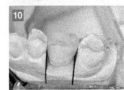
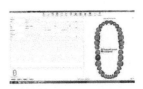

Procedure

1. Create the work record in the software package detailing the type and position of the restoration, the opposing dentition and the type of inter-occlusal record (Figure 4.27.2).

Figure 4.27.2

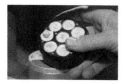

Figure 4.27.3

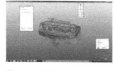

Figure 4.27.4

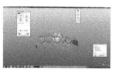

Figure 4.27.5

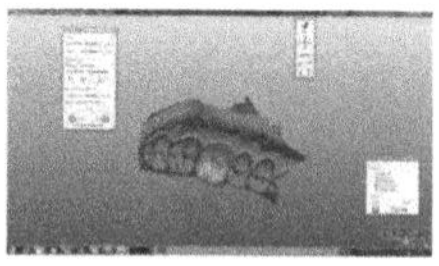

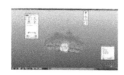

Figure 4.27.6

Figure 4.27.7

Figure 4.27.8

2. Scan the model by inserting it into the holder and working through the scanning wizard. A separate scan of the die has been carried out here to ensure the margin data is captured in the interproximal areas (Figure 4.27.3).

3. Scan the opposing dentition by either using an occlusal registration as shown, or by scanning the opposing teeth and carrying out a correlation scan (Figure 4.27.4).

4. Using the design package, work through the wizard to create a full contour restoration (Figure 4.27.5).

5. Carry out a cut-back in the desired areas (Figures 4.27.6 and 4.27.7).

6. Save the restoration design and export to the CAM software for milling (Figure 4.27.8).

7. Mill as in Section 4.26.

4.28 Producing a bridge substructure

Introduction

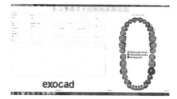

Figure 4.28.1

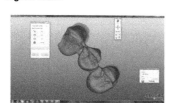

Figure 4.28.2

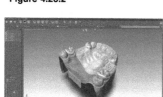

Figure 4.29.1

Bridge frameworks may be produced with or without the opposing dentition, as for the single-unit restoration examples shown above. In the following example a bridge framework is being designed using the cut-back technique.

The difference is ensuring that the correct teeth are chosen as abutment or pontic accordingly, and that the connectors are chosen at the outset of the design process (Figures 4.28.1 and 4.28.2).

4.29 Removable Partial Denture Design

Introduction

In this example, the Dental Wings scanner and software is being used to create a CAD RPD framework for a CoCr framework. The design can be used to either mill, selective laser sinter or 3D print in wax for casting (Figure 4.29.1).

The method for scanning is similar to that described above with the exception that the palatal data must be included.

Work safety

The CAD–CAM systems have failsafe measures to prevent injury (which should not be tampered with). Dust and eye protection should be used when trimming die stone and the substructure material.

You will need:

- A model produced in a scannable die stone (or powder spray)
- Material to be machined.

Basic procedure

1. A bite registration is taken, and the working and opposing (antagonist) models scanned in (as for single-unit restorations – see Section 4.27).

2. At the stage where the margins are entered, the pontics are also outlined on the alveolar ridge.

3. Each unit is designed to full contour, using the opposing dentition.

4. The bridge framework is reduced (either partially or fully).

5. The connectors between abutment and pontic may be selected and adjusted for position and size.

6. Bridge frameworks should be machined from the highest strength materials, either zirconia or laser-sintered metal.

7. The framework can also be produced in the dental laboratory by casting the substructure after milling it in a wax substitute.

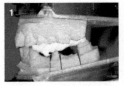
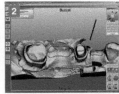
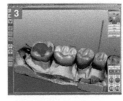
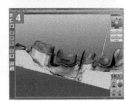
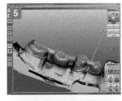
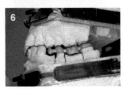
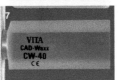

Extended information

Methods of Advanced Manufacture

Currently, the advanced manufacture (AM) of dental restorations, prostheses or models is dominated by subtractive computer numerical controlled (CNC) machining technology and additive wax deposition modelling (WDM), the latter relying on traditional lost wax casting technology for production of the final part. However, a number of other more energy-efficient and less wasteful direct additive layered manufacturing processes are becoming more commonly used with each able to build a three-dimensional part from a number of polymer resin or metal powders thereby providing greater consistency in manufacture whilst achieving a reduction in both time and cost.

Computer Numerical Controlled (CNC) Machining

CNC 'refers to machining process which is operated using automated computer control, as opposed to manually by an operator'. Generally they consist of a platform that moves in both the X-axis (horizontal) and the Y-axis (vertical) and cutting tool(s) that move along the Z-axis (depth). Depending upon the CNC machine, these may have three or five machining axes of movement, with each axis indicating the number of directions any burr or cutting tool may approach.

Continued over

In each case, a customised CAM programme defining the 3D geometry of the part is created and uploaded to the CNC machine, which then interprets the data for processing. However, these software command files differ, with many earlier dental CAD–CAM systems providing dedicated or 'closed source' files which may only be accessed for manufacture with similar proprietary software, whereas more recent 'open source' software provides greater compatibility as it uses a standardised computer language, for example, 'stl programme commands' which may be uploaded and recognised by CNC machines of independent in-house or out-sourced manufacturers.

Depending upon the part's design these 3D geometric shapes may be machined from a variety of dental materials, including metals, ceramics, composites, plastics, or machining waxes recommended for the lost wax process. A block of the required material is either manually or automatically attached to the machine-table in order to maintain a fixed datum position throughout the machining process. On completion, all machined connectors between the final part and the remaining portion of the block require separation prior to finishing, along with the need for consideration as to waste management handling in order to lower the environmental impact.

Other considerations

Advantages:

- Generally a good range of materials available

- Open systems enable machining by independent manufacturers

- Produces parts with superior strength and surface finish compared to additive manufacture.

Disadvantages:

- Closed systems restrict access for manufacture.

- Considerable waste material to manage or dispose of adding to both cost and carbon footprint.

- Difficulty in machining highly complex or undercut surfaces.

- May require experienced programmers and machinists, which can add to cost.

- Requires substantial connectors to main body of material to avoid distortion and maintain datum position during machining.

- Time consuming by comparison to some other methods of advanced manufacture.

- Where soft plastic and wax materials are used wall thickness needs consideration.

- Where a wax part is machined for traditional casting processes, recognised casting problems still exist.

Continued over

Metal-Laser Sintering, Laser Melting and Electron Beam Melting (LS, LM and EBM)

Although laser sintering (LS), laser melting (LM) and electron beam melting (EBM) have been used for some time in the medical field to produce fully dense metallic parts, their introduction into dentistry has been more recent. One area where these processes are gaining popularity is the direct manufacture of single and multiple-unit metal copings for dental restorations, thereby avoiding the recognised problems associated with traditional lost wax casting technology. For similar reasons, some manufacturers are currently evaluating these technologies for the manufacture of RPD metal frameworks; however, economic volumes, manufacturing times and/or conformity with Medical Devices Directive are difficulties yet to be fully addressed.

Although these melting processes are similar, with each fully melting the metal powder in thin (approximately 20–100 µm) layers to directly create the required part their energy source differs, with LS and LM using high-powered laser, whereas EBM uses an electron beam.

The manufacturing process for each requires a build platform which allows both for anchorage of the part and heat dissipation during manufacture. As with other additive layering processes the extracted 3D CAD models are checked and support structures introduced before orientation and nesting within the build volume, thereby providing maximum productivity. In the LS and LM process the chamber is back filled with argon or nitrogen to give an inert process environment, whereas in the case of EBM the build process is carried out under vacuum. However, in either case the resultant materials that are produced are fully dense and void free, with mechanical properties mid-way between a cast and wrought material. On completion of AM manufacturing, all support structures need to be removed and any necessary surface finishing undertaken. Currently the laser process manufactures a more accurate component with some production parts manufactured down to 20 µm.

Importantly, there is little waste material to manage when using these additive layering processes when compared to CNC machining processes, as the majority of the supporting powder is collected for reuse.

Other considerations (laser melting – LM)

Advantages:

- Able to produce parts with undercuts and complex geometries.

- Can produce accurate parts with detailed resolution and good surface quality.

- Although the process can work with pure or reactive metals (e.g. Ti) as it is undertaken in an inert atmosphere, in some cases the addition of alloying materials may be required.

- Eliminates problems of lost wax casting by direct manufacture of metal parts.

- Fully melts the powdered metal particles into a homogenous mass.

- Little waste material to manage or dispose of, thereby minimising cost and carbon footprint.

Continued over

- Rapidly and accurately produces a functional custom-designed metal part making the process cost effective.

Disadvantages:

- Equipment is not generally available in commercial dental laboratories or hospitals.

- Currently when considering dental processes a limited range of powdered metals available.

- Insufficient manufacturing volumes for some dental appliances.

- Not all materials or processes currently conform to EU's regulations on the manufacture of Medical Devices Directive.

- Requires post processing to remove metallic support structures.

Other considerations (electron beam melting – EBM)

Advantages:

- Able to produce parts with undercuts and complex geometries.

- The parts produced are less accurate with relatively poor surface quality.

- Although the process can be used with pure or reactive metals being undertaken in an inert atmosphere, it is limited to Ti64 and CoCr.

- Where large components may be required EBM is significantly faster than LM, making the process more cost effective.

- Eliminates problems of lost wax casting by direct manufacture of metal parts.

- Fully melts the powdered metal particles into a homogenous mass.

- Little waste material to manage or dispose of, thereby minimising cost and carbon footprint.

- Produces void-free and extremely strong metal parts.

Disadvantages:

- Equipment is not generally available in commercial dental laboratories or hospitals.

- Currently a limited range of powdered metals is available.

- Insufficient manufacturing volumes for some dental appliances.

- Not all materials or processes currently conform to EU's regulations on the manufacture of Medical Devices Directive.

- Parts are less accurate than laser.

- Requires post processing to remove metallic support structures.

Procedure

1. Create the work record in the software package detailing the type of appliance (Figure 4.29.2).

2. Scan the model by inserting it into the holder and working through the scanning wizard (Figure 4.29.3).

3. Using the design package, work through the wizard to

    (a) create a path of insertion (Figure 4.29.4).

    (b) block out undercuts (Figure 4.29.5).

    (c) adjust blocking out to accommodate clasps (Figure 4.29.6).

    (d) add Occlusal rests, clasps and reciprocation (Figures 4.29.7 and 4.29.8).

    (e) design saddle area and connectors (Figure 4.29.9).

    (f) add any minor connectors and finishing edges (Figure 4.29.10).

4. Save the design and export to the CAM software for milling or printing (Figures 4.29.1 and 4.29.11).

5. The design may now be made using an appropriate processing method.

4.30 Implant-supported prosthodontics

Introduction to implant-supported prosthodontics

Implants are beyond the scope of this book, and this section outlines the main principles. Where teeth have been lost, osseointegrated (osseo meaning bone) dental implants may provide support for a restoration (Figure 4.30.1).

Alternatively, several implants may be used to support a denture (Figure 4.30.2).

There are many different dental implant systems, but the principles are common to them all. The fixture (made from titanium, Figure 4.30.3) is surgically implanted into the alveolar bone.

To allow a restoration to be made, an impression is taken. An abutment is placed on the fixture and an impression taken of the dentition to incorporate the abutment. This is sent to the laboratory where a fixture replica is positioned on the abutment (Figure 4.30.4).

A model is cast and the fixture replica is incorporated into the model (Figure 4.30.5), allowing the technician to produce a restoration.

The abutment is attached to the fixture by a screw, and a restoration is either cemented or screwed to the abutment (Figure 4.30.6).

Implant retained prostheses are either permanently fixed in place either using screws or are cemented (Figures 4.30.2 and 4.30.6) or they are patient removable (Figures 4.30.7), the latter being held in place by 'press-stud' type attachments that have a male part attached to the head of the implant and a female part embedded in the fitting surface of the denture (Figure 4.30.8).

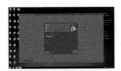
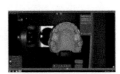
Figure 4.29.2   **Figure 4.29.3**

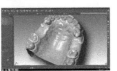
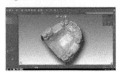
Figure 4.29.4   **Figure 4.29.5**

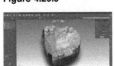
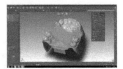
Figure 4.29.6   **Figure 4.29.7**

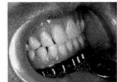
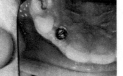
Figure 4.29.8   **Figure 4.29.9**

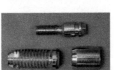
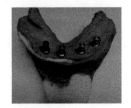
Figure 4.29.10   **Figure 4.29.11**

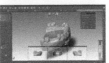
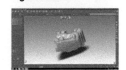
Figure 4.30.1   **Figure 4.30.2**

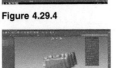
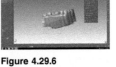
Figure 4.30.3

Figure 4.30.4

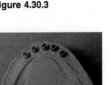
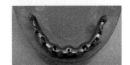
Figure 4.30.5   **Figure 4.30.6**

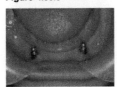
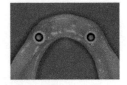
Figure 4.30.7

Figure 4.30.8

Chapter 5 | ORTHODONTICS

5.1 Introduction to orthodontics

Orthodontics is the area of dentistry that concentrates on the correction of malocclusions. This includes correction of the way in which the teeth are aligned or the correction of the skeletal relationship between the upper and lower dental arches. The aim of orthodontics, therefore, is to achieve perfect occlusion.

Modern orthodontics is based in the main on the work of two people, Edward Angle, whose classification of malocclusion is universally used, and Lawrence Andrews, whose 'six keys to occlusion' re-defined Angle's work.

Indications for orthodontic treatment

The use of removable orthodontic appliances has reduced somewhat in recent years due to the advances that have been made in fixed appliance therapy. However, there is a role for removable appliances as an adjunct to fixed appliance treatment and in specially selected patients in whom the limitations of the removable appliance are not exceeded. They are particularly effective in mixed dentition malocclusions, as space maintainers and for retainer appliances following treatment with fixed appliances.

Benefits of orthodontic treatment

1. Aesthetics

People's appearance is important to them, as is the need to conform to what is regarded as normal within their culture. A dental appearance that is outside of what is felt to be normal may lead to a feeling of low self-esteem. Treatment of a patient with a malocclusion that is causing them to experience low self-esteem will give greater confidence and a feeling of well-being about their dental appearance.

2. Function

A malocclusion may interfere with the correct function of speech. The most common problem is the pronunciation of the letter 'S'.

3. Dental health

Overcrowding of the teeth may lead to caries due to the inability to keep the teeth clean in an effective way.

Disadvantages of orthodontic treatment

1. Root resorption

This can happen if the bone of the palatal vault does not respond to the movement of, for example, an incisor, and therefore acts to restrict its movement; this may then lead to resorption of the incisor apex instead of the bone.

Basics of Dental Technology: A Step By Step Approach, Second Edition.
Tony Johnson, David G. Patrick, Christopher W. Stokes, David G. Wildgoose and Duncan J. Wood.
© 2016 John Wiley & Sons, Ltd. Published 2016 by John Wiley & Sons, Ltd.
Companion Website: www.wiley.com/go/johnson/basicsdentaltechnology

2. Loss of periodontal support

If too great a force is applied to a tooth, the blood capillaries are occluded and cells in the periodontal ligament die. This area is then structureless or 'hyalinised'. The hyaline material consists of compressed collagen.

3. Decalcification

When fixed appliances are removed, sometimes white spot lesions are noted in the enamel of the tooth underneath where the bracket was bonded; these are due to decalcification of the enamel.

4. Soft tissue damage

The soft tissues can be injured and painful and sore areas can occur under wires or the baseplate of an appliance. However, these problems are generally dealt with fairly easily.

5.2 Classification of malocclusions

Angle's classification of malocclusion

Known as the 'father of orthodontics', the American orthodontist Edward Hartley Angle (1855–1930) produced a classification for the different forms of malocclusion.

Class I

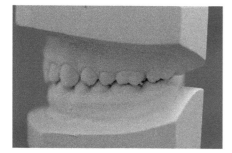

Figure 5.2.1

This is the normal anteroposterior relationship of the maxilla to the mandible (no skeletal discrepancy) (Figure 5.2.1), characterised by the mesio-buccal cusp of the first upper permanent molar occluding in the mesio-buccal groove of the lower first permanent molar.

A Class I relationship is usually accepted as normal and although there are no skeletal discrepancies there may be some problems that can be corrected with removable appliances. The use of a removable appliance will depend on the problem and whether a removable appliance can deliver the kind of tooth movement that is required. Often simple tooth movements can be achieved easily with active components such as springs (sometimes along with necessary tooth extractions).

Class II

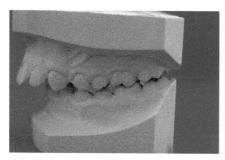

Figure 5.2.2

This is a posterior relationship of the mandible to the maxilla. The mesio-buccal cusp of the first upper permanent molar occludes mesial to the mesio-buccal groove of the lower first permanent molar.

Division 1: The maxillary incisors are proclined, giving rise to a 'buck-toothed' appearance (Figure 5.2.2).

Division 2: The upper centrals are proclined and the upper laterals are retroclined; there is also a deep overbite associated with this division (Figure 5.2.3).

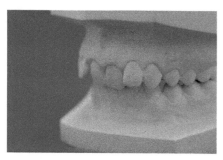

Figure 5.2.3

Where there is no skeletal discrepancy but the upper incisors are very proclined, the use of a removable appliance can achieve very good results. However, where the overjet is because of a skeletal problem, functional appliance therapy is usually needed followed by a course of fixed appliance treatment.

Class III

This is an anterior relationship of the mandible to the maxilla. The mesio-buccal cusp of the upper first permanent molar occludes distal to the mesio-buccal groove of the lower first permanent molar (Figure 5.2.4).

To correct a Class III malocclusion satisfactorily with removable appliances, there should only be a mild Class III relationship or ideally a Class I skeletal relationship with the incisors being in a Class III relationship.

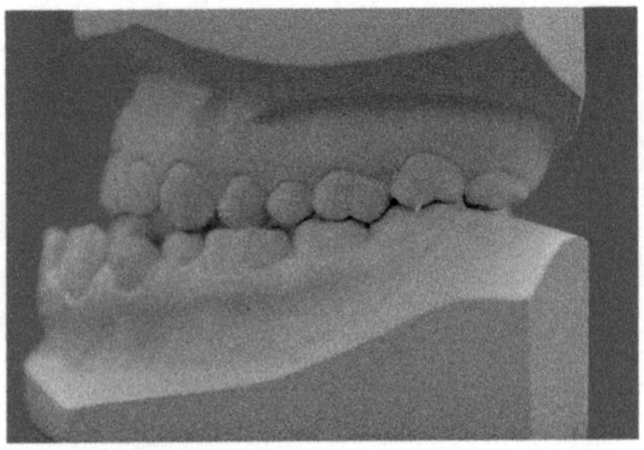

Figure 5.2.4

Andrew's six keys to occlusion

(1) Molar relationship: the distal surface of the disto-buccal cusp of the upper first permanent molar occludes with the mesial surface of the mesio-buccal cusp of the lower second permanent molar.

(2) Crown angulation (mesio-distal tip): the gingival portion of each crown is distal to the incisal portion and varies with each tooth type.

(3) Crown inclination (labio-lingual, bucco-lingual): anterior teeth should be at a sufficient angulation to prevent over-eruption. The upper posterior teeth should have a constant lingual tip that is similar from the canines to the second premolars and then increased in the molars. In the lower posterior teeth, the lingual tip increases progressively from the canines to the molar.

(4) No rotations.

(5) No spaces.

(6) Flat occlusal planes.

Orthodontic treatment falls into one of two areas: 'camouflage' and 'modification'. Treatment goals have to be decided on early and may possibly be a compromise between the patient's most favoured outcome, which might purely be one of aesthetics where as an orthodontist may wish to achieve perfect occlusion.

Designing orthodontic appliances is a team exercise involving the orthodontist and technician. In order to do so, the technician should understand the concepts of anchorage, retention and tooth movement.

5.3 Theory of tooth movement

When force is applied to the crown of a tooth it will move slightly within the surrounding periodontal ligament. Then, because of the areas of compression that have been set up, the tooth will move to a new position in the mouth if the force is applied over a sufficient length of time. There are three kinds of movement that one can expect: tipping, bodily movement and rotation about the long axis. Tipping of a tooth is the only kind of movement that a removable appliance can achieve, bodily moving a tooth is only possible with fixed appliances and rotations can be achieved with removable appliances if managed closely.

Removable appliances

A removable appliance is one that can be easily removed from the mouth; however, this does not mean that they are for part-time wear.

The use of removable orthodontic appliances has fallen due to the limited range of movements that can be achieved with them and consequently the popularity of fixed appliance therapies. However, they are still required in the form of retainers and functional appliances used in combination with fixed appliance therapy. In addition, they can be used for simple movements such as tipping a tooth, which are easily achieved with them.

Anchorage

Anchorage is an important consideration when moving teeth and should not be confused with retention (how an appliance is held in the mouth). Anchorage is the resistance to movement by the teeth when an orthodontic force is applied.

Incorrect provision of anchorage for an appliance will allow the tooth that is being moved to stay where it is, and the 'anchoring' teeth to move.

Removable appliances often rely on intra-maxillary traction, where anchorage is obtained from within the same arch. Reciprocal anchorage is also possible, that is, the force of movement of two teeth, or groups of teeth, cancels each other out. A simple example is that of closing a diastema. Other than in these cases, the reactionary force generated to move a tooth is distributed to other teeth such that they can resist movement.

Retention

The term retention is used in orthodontics to mean two things:

(1) The means by which an appliance is held in the mouth

(2) The means by which the teeth are retained in their new position after movement.

A removable appliance is held in the mouth in two ways. Firstly, by using clasps in tooth undercuts and, secondly, by means of the baseplate which may also use undercut areas on the palatal aspect of the teeth and in the same way as a denture, use the close fit of the plate and saliva on the palate to create cohesion between the appliance and the soft tissues.

Maintaining teeth in their new position is carried out using retainers. Either Hawley or Essix-type retainers can be used and do the job equally well. Essix-type retainers are worn for much less time, generally at night; and as they are virtually invisible when in place they are becoming increasingly popular.

Casting working model ▸ Component construction ▸ Removable appliance construction

5.4 Basic wire bending techniques

Introduction

A number of basic bends are used in the construction of orthodontic appliances.

Using pliers

You will need:
- Adams pliers
- Spring-forming pliers
- Wire cutters
- 0.7 mm stainless steel wire

The pliers should only be used as a vice to grip the wire; nearly all wire bending is done with the thumb and index finger.

Straightening wire

Most wire is supplied on reels; therefore, once a length of wire has been cut, it will have a pronounced curve. In most cases the wire will require straightening before a component can be made.

(1) Hold the wire tightly with the Adams pliers at one end so that it curves towards you (Figure 5.4.1).

(2) Pull your thumb and index finger along the wire applying pressure against the curve of the wire (Figure 5.4.2).

(3) Repeat if necessary to fully straighten the wire (Figure 5.4.3).

Soft curves

When forming soft curves the wire does not require straightening; the curve that is already present can be exaggerated to help form the curve. This is done for components such as the labial bow.

(1) Hold the wire in both hands and bend the ends towards each other.

(2) Alternatively, use one hand to increase the curve by 'squashing' the wire between the fingers and the thumb (Figure 5.4.4).

Right-angled bends

(1) Firmly grip the wire between the tips of the Adams pliers (Figure 5.4.5).

(2) Bend the wire at 90° to the pliers with the thumb close to the pliers and exerting a lot of pressure to form a tight bend (Figure 5.4.6).

Acute-angled bends

These types of bend are demanding on your fingers and require a firm grip on the pliers.

(1) Hold the wire so that it emerges over the tips of the Adams pliers (Figure 5.4.7).

(2) With the thumb close to the pliers, bend the wire over the beaks of the pliers (Figure 5.4.8).

Coils and loops

To make coils and loops, found in springs and labial bows, 'spring-forming' pliers must be used. Making uniform coils and loops takes practice but is simple once the technique has been mastered. The wire should be bent around the conical beak of the spring-forming pliers and constantly moved so that the square beak does not hinder the process.

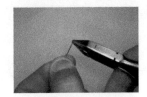

Figure 5.4.1

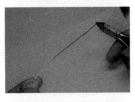

Figure 5.4.2

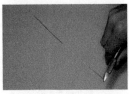

Figure 5.4.3

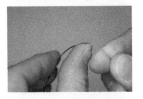

Figure 5.4.4

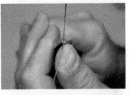

Figure 5.4.5

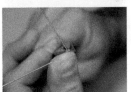

Figure 5.4.6

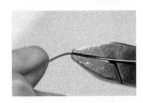

Figure 5.4.7

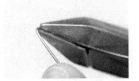

Figure 5.4.8

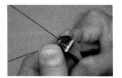

Figure 5.4.9

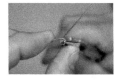

Figure 5.4.10

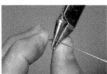

Figure 5.4.11

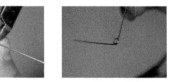

Figure 5.4.12

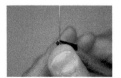

Figure 5.4.13

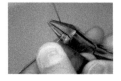

Figure 5.4.14

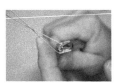

Figure 5.4.15

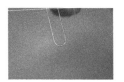

Figure 5.4.16

(1) Push the wire with the thumb around the conical beak until a 'U' has been formed at the tip of the pliers (Figure 5.4.9).

(2) Take one side of this 'U' over the other ensuring that the two wires stay in firm contact with each other and continue to bend until a full circle has been made (Figure 5.4.10).

(3) Take the coil off the pliers and put it back on from the other side (Figure 5.4.11).

(4) Continue to push the wire round the pliers until both sides are parallel (Figure 5.4.12).

Large radius bends

(1) The wire is held in the pliers in the same way as for the right-angled bend (Figure 5.4.13).

(2) Instead of bending the wire with the thumb close to the pliers, the thumb and index finger bend the wire a small distance away from the pliers (Figure 5.4.14).

(3) Continue to push the wire round the pliers (Figure 5.4.15) until the bend is complete (Figure 5.4.16).

5.5 Making passive components

Passive components are the parts of a removable appliance that are responsible for holding the appliance in the mouth and holding the teeth that are not being moved.

5.6 Producing ball-ended clasps

Casting working model ＞ Component construction ＞ Removable appliance construction

You will need:

- Adams pliers
- Wire cutters
- Pre-formed ball-ended clasps, either 0.8 or 0.9 mm
- 2B pencil

Work safety

Safety glasses should be worn when handling orthodontic wires.

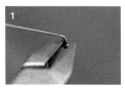

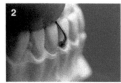

Introduction

Ball-ended clasps are quick and easy to make. They are bought pre-formed so just need fitting to the model. The ball end fits low down in between two teeth and rests on the gingival margin.

Basic procedure

1. Hold the ball in the pliers and make a right-angled bend as close to the ball as possible.

2. Place the ball in between the teeth where the clasp is to be positioned so that the long wire part of the clasp rests against the contact point between the two teeth, and then mark that point with the pencil.

Continued over

3. From this pencil mark the wire should then be adapted to the contours of the teeth and model, making sure that it is kept out of the way of the opposing model.

4. To finish the clasp on the palatal or lingual surface make a right-angled bend to aid its retention in the acrylic baseplate.

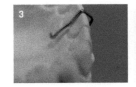
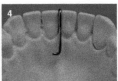

5.7 The Adams clasp

Adams clasps are the most widely used clasp on removable appliances, particularly on molars and premolars (Figure 5.7.1). There are other clasps that can and sometimes are used but the Adams is the most versatile.

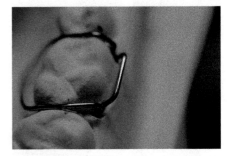

Figure 5.7.1

You will need:

- Adams pliers
- Wire cutters
- 0.7 mm stainless steel wire
- 2B pencil
- Ash No. 10 carver

Basic procedure

1. Survey the model (by eye) to look for available undercuts.

2. If no undercut is available, 'pockets' should be cut into the gingival margin into which the clasp will engage.

3. Carve the pockets making sure that they are not too deep and that they follow the contour of the unerupted buccal surface of the tooth to be clasped.

4. Cut a piece of 0.7 mm wire about 10 cm long and straighten. Near the centre make a 90° bend.

5. Place this bend on the inside of one of the pockets.

6. Mark the wire where it touches the inside of the other pocket.

7. At the mark make another 90° bend in the same plane as the first. This will form the 'bridge' of the clasp. It must be made the correct length.

8. Check that the two bends are 90°.

Continued over

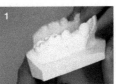
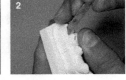
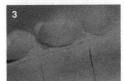
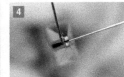
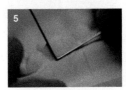
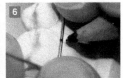
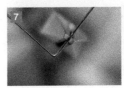
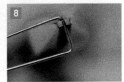

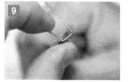
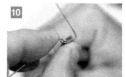
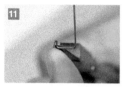
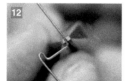
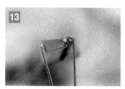
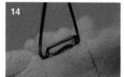
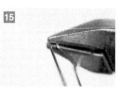
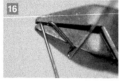
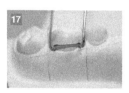
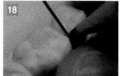
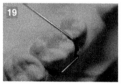
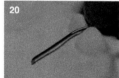
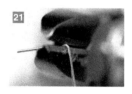
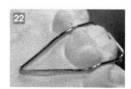

9. Form the arrowheads by holding the wire so that the bridge is horizontal and the two ends are vertical. Grip one of the vertical pieces with the tips of the Adams pliers, 2–3 mm from the bridge.

10. Bend the wire through 90° away from the other wire arm.

11. Continue to bend the wire down but at the same time bring it around in front of the beak of the pliers.

12. An arrowhead should now have formed – a small 'u' shape – and both sides must be parallel; the arrowhead must be 3–4 mm long.

13. Repeat the process for the other side so that there are two arrowheads of the same size and shape. They both must be 90° to the bridge when viewed from the buccal aspect and 45° to the bridge when viewed from the gingival aspect.

14. The two arrowheads must fit exactly into the pockets.

15. From the buccal aspect grip the mesial arrowhead in the tips of the Adams pliers just below halfway up the arrowhead – as the bend must be well below the bridge.

16. With the thumb close to the pliers bend the wire across the pliers and then pull the wire round so that it is at 90° to the bridge.

17. If all the bends are in the right places and at the right angles when the clasp is placed on the tooth the mesial part will contact the tooth to be clasped and the adjacent tooth such that the rest of the clasp is at 45° to the tooth; this angle must be maintained for the clasp to function correctly.

18. Where the wire contacts the tooth it should be marked with a pencil to indicate where the next bend is to be made.

19. The wire should now be fitted to follow the contour of the embrasure between the teeth – it must not be high over the occlusion.

20. When fitting the wire in the palate it must be straight (if possible) and a gap of about 0.5–1 mm must be present between it and the model.

21. Bend and cut a small right-angled bend at the end of the wire to aid retention in the baseplate.

22. Once the mesial side is done the same process is repeated with the distal side. The distal wire must be carried forward to meet the mesial wire, so that the baseplate can be trimmed away from the soft palate.

Casting working model > Component construction > Removable appliance construction

5.8 Producing a southend clasp

Southend clasps are used on removable appliances that need a clasp in the anterior region. They are fitted close to the gingival margin of either the two central incisors or a central and a lateral incisor, and because of this they are relatively unobtrusive (Figure 5.8.1).

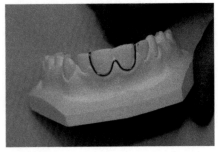

Figure 5.8.1

Basic procedure

1. Cut a piece of 0.7 mm wire (10 cm long) and without straightening it out make a very acute-angled 'V' shaped bend in the centre. This will then lie in between the two teeth that are being clasped.

2. Hold this in place on the model and note where the wire leaves the surface of one of the teeth either with a pencil or by using the pliers.

3. Bend the wire at this point such that it will conform to the contour of the labial surface of the tooth.

4. Check the bends frequently against the model.

5. Repeat this process until the wire fits all the way around the gingival margin and the wire is pointing down the tooth contacting closely between the tooth being clasped and the one adjacent to it.

6. Mark the wire at the embrasure and make an acute bend so that the wire will follow the contour of the embrasure and lie directly in between the clasped tooth and the adjacent one. (A bend may have to be made to keep the end of the wire from touching the palate, allowing the fit of the wire to be checked.)

7. Fit the wire to the palate, keeping it as straight as possible, leaving a gap of 0.5–1 mm between it and the model.

8. Repeat this process with the other half of the clasp.

9. Make both palatal tags symmetrical, taking into consideration other components.

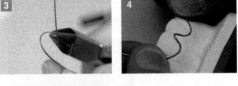

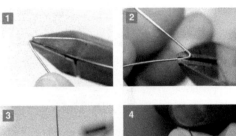

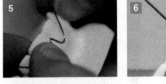

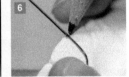

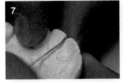

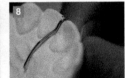

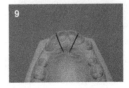

5.9 Active appliances

An active removable appliance incorporates one or more of the following components: spring, screw, elastic or labial bow.

Springs

Springs can move teeth in two different ways:

(1) Along the line of the arch, either anteriorly or posteriorly using palatal finger springs

(2) Into alignment in the arch, either palatally or labially/buccally.

Springs will do one or the other of these movements but not both so if a tooth needs to be moved posteriorly and palatally two different spring components will have to be used.

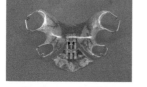

Figure 5.9.1

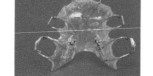

Figure 5.9.2

Screws

As an alternative to using springs to move teeth, there are a very wide variety of screws that can be incorporated into the appliance. They deliver the force required to move a tooth or group of teeth via the acrylic baseplate. The patient activates the screw usually once a week. A high force is generated initially, but this force soon reduces as the tooth/teeth move. Screws can be used for all manner of tooth movements, and appliance designs to accomplish these are shown below.

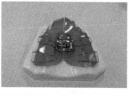

Figure 5.9.3

- Pushing anterior teeth over the bite (Figure 5.9.1)
- Closing a diastema, or pushing distally or mesially (Figure 5.9.2)
- Expanding the arch (Figure 5.9.3).

It is possible that for every type of tooth movement possible there is a screw or combination of screws that can be used.

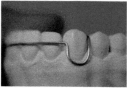

Figure 5.9.4

Elastics

Elastics are generally used with removable appliances for intermaxillary traction or for more localised tooth movement where a hook or button is bonded to a tooth and the elastic is attached to this on one end and to the appliance at the other to provide the force required.

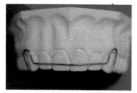

Figure 5.9.5

Labial bows

A labial bow (Figures 5.9.4 and 5.9.5) may be used passively, for example, in a retainer, or it can be used for the movement of teeth – retracting the incisors. The most common type of bow used for this purpose, particularly if the overjet is large, is a Roberts retractor (Figure 5.9.6).

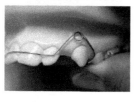

Figure 5.9.6

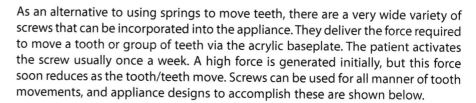

5.10 Palatal finger spring (guarded)

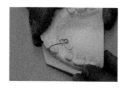

Figure 5.10.1

These are made from 0.5 or 0.6 mm wire; 0.6 mm wire springs are activated by a smaller amount to give the same amount of force. A coil is incorporated into the spring to increase its length and consequently its flexibility. The coil should lie on the opposite side to the spring arm such that when it is 'activated' to move a tooth, the spring is unwinding (Figure 5.10.1).

You will need:

- Adams pliers
- Spring-forming pliers
- Wire cutters
- 0.5 mm stainless steel wire – 6 cm length
- 2B pencil
- Wax knife
- Modelling wax
- Ash No. 5 carver
- Bunsen burner

Work safety

Safety glasses should be worn when handling orthodontic wires.

Basic procedure

1. Determine the intended path of tooth movement, and then mark with a pencil the point on the tooth where the spring will make contact. Draw a line on the model perpendicular to the path of tooth movement through the middle of the crown of the tooth.

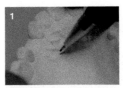
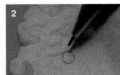

2. Draw the coil on the model at least 10 mm from the tooth; it should lie on the perpendicular drawn in step 1.

3. Straighten out about 100 mm of wire and make a coil with an internal diameter of 3 mm in the centre of the wire, and finish such that the two wires that emerge from the coil are roughly parallel. Ensure that the wire that will form the spring arm is emerging from the bottom of the coil.

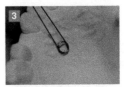
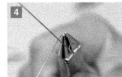

4. Form the guard by making an 80° bend in the guard wire mid-way between the coil and the tooth. This wire should then pass under the spring arm so that it will lie flat against the model and span the full extent of the intended path of movement of the tooth. Finish the guard with a 90° bend parallel with the spring arm, keeping clear of the model.

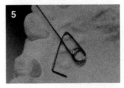
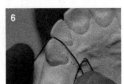

5. Fit the spring to the model, and avoid the use of pliers as soft gentle curves are required.

6. Adapt the spring arm to the tooth that is being moved. It should lie well below the embrasure and extend a few millimetres down the labial surface of the tooth.

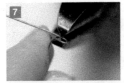
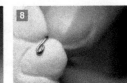

7. Finish the end with a small eyelet that lies flat to the labial surface of the tooth ensuring that there are no sharp ends of wire. Bend the wire around the tip of the pliers making sure to pass the wire in front of the beaks to get a very tight radius bend.

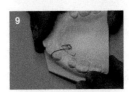

8. Cut off the long end and squeeze the eyelet together using Adams pliers.

9. The spring arm should be straight unless a bend is required to make correct contact with the tooth.

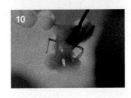

10. Wax in place and 'box out', using a small amount of molten wax on the spring to hold it in place, and add more wax in increments until the working parts of the spring are all encased in wax.

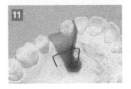

11. Trim and smooth, leaving enough room for the spring to function.

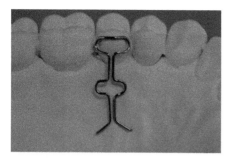

Figure 5.11.1

5.11 Making a T-spring

T-springs are made from 0.5 mm wire and are only vaguely 'T' shaped. They are used on premolars and molars and fit right up to the tip of the palatal cusp (Figure 5.11.1).

You will need:

- Adams pliers
- Spring-forming pliers
- Wire cutters
- 0.5 mm stainless steel wire – 6 cm length
- 2B pencil
- Wax knife
- Modelling wax
- Ash No. 5 carver
- Bunsen burner

Basic procedure

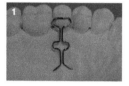
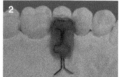

1. Straighten out the wire, and then make the spring, as pictured, making sure that the part that engages the crown of the tooth is not too wide.

2. The length of the spring should be about 1 cm plus the tags that hold it in the acrylic.

Impression → Casting working model → Component construction → Removable appliance construction

5.12 Double cantilever or Z-spring

This is an adaptation of the palatal finger spring and is used for moving a tooth labially. It has two coils, hence double cantilever, and therefore can move the tooth in a more controlled way (Figure 5.12.1). For example, if a central incisor is slightly rotated, the spring can push the tooth so that it appears to de-rotate; the spring would have to be used in conjunction with a labial bow to do this.

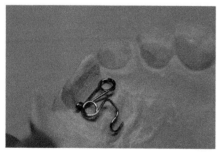

Figure 5.12.1

You will need:

- Adams pliers
- Spring-forming pliers
- Wire cutters
- 0.5 mm stainless steel wire
- 2B pencil
- Wax knife
- Modelling wax
- Ash No. 5 carver
- Bunsen burner

Basic procedure

1. Make an eyelet in one end of the straightened piece of wire. Bend the wire around the tip of the pliers, making sure to pass the wire in front of the beaks to get a very acute radius bend, cut off the long end and then squeeze together using Adams pliers. Place this eyelet on the mesial edge of the tooth to be moved and mark on the wire the distal edge.

2. At the pencil mark make a small coil bending away from the part that engages the tooth so that the free end comes from the top of the coil.

3. Once parallel with the part that engages the tooth, make another coil opposite the eyelet, bending the wire away from the eyelet so that it points back towards the other coil. Make a mark on this piece of wire between the two coils and make a 90° bend away from the spring to form the tag.

4. Make a bend in the tag for retention in the acrylic.

5. The spring should now be concertinaed together, ready for its activation in the appliance. Hold one of the coils in the spring-forming pliers and push the other coil towards the pliers.

6. Once the spring is made it can be waxed in place and 'boxed out'. This means that a small amount of molten wax is placed on the spring to hold it in place on the model.

7. More wax is added incrementally until the working parts of the spring are all encased in wax.

8. This must then be trimmed and made as neat and as smooth as possible whilst leaving enough room for the spring to function.

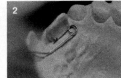
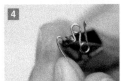
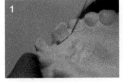
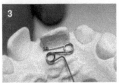
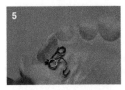
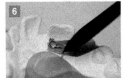
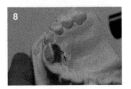
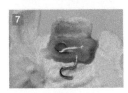

5.13 Buccal canine retractor

Buccal canine retractors are used to retract canines that are positioned buccally, and push them palatally into the line of the arch (Figure 5.13.1). They are usually made from 0.5 mm wire that is supported and strengthened by stainless steel tubing. The 0.7 mm without the tubing may be used; however, the force it delivers is high and better results are achieved with low forces when moving teeth. There are several different ways the retractor may contact tooth; the most popular is described.

The coil should lie in between the tooth being retracted and the mesial surface of the adjacent tooth towards which the tooth is being retracted. The coil should also be 3–4 mm short of the sulcus.

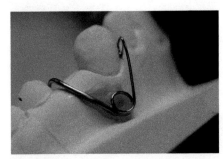

Figure 5.13.1

You will need:

- Adams pliers
- Spring-forming pliers
- Wire cutters
- 0.5 mm stainless steel wire
- 0.5 mm internal diameter stainless steel tubing
- 2B pencil
- Wax knife
- Modelling wax
- Ash No 5 carver
- Bunsen burner
- Cut-off disc
- Micromotor

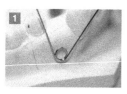
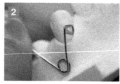
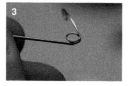
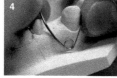
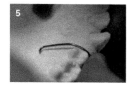
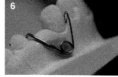

Basic procedure

1. Straighten out the 0.5 mm wire. Make a coil with an internal diameter of about 3 mm in the centre of the wire and hold against the model in the correct position and mark the wire where the end is to be made that will engage the tooth.

2. A 'golf club' end is made to engage low down on the canine nearer to the gingival margin than the tip of the tooth.

3. Using a cut-off disc bevel one end of a 5 cm piece of 0.5 mm internal diameter stainless steel tube so that it appears similar to the sharpened end of a pencil. Slide the tubing onto the wire right up to the coil.

4. Bend the tubed wire to fit the model, keeping away from where the tooth is to be retracted and below the height of the occlusion.

5. Put a small right-angled bend in the end of the tag for retention.

6. Seal in place with hot wax.

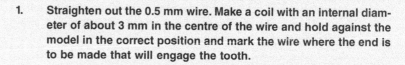

Impression → Casting working model → Component construction → Removable appliance construction

5.14 The Roberts retractor

The Roberts retractor has two buccal canine retractors that are joined by a labial bow (Figure 5.14.1). This retractor is technically demanding to produce; however, it helps achieve good results when reducing a large overjet.

The arch is placed in the incisal third of the incisor teeth and starts from 2 mm from the distal edge of the laterals.

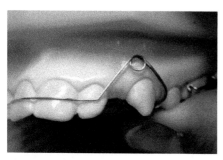

Figure 5.14.1

You will need:

- Adams pliers
- Spring-forming pliers
- Wire cutters
- 0.5 mm stainless steel wire
- Two 5 cm lengths of 0.5 mm internal diameter bevelled stainless steel tubing 2B pencil
- Wax knife
- Modelling wax
- Ash No. 5 carver
- Bunsen burner
- Cut-off disc
- Micromotor

Basic procedure

1. Firstly the arch should be made to conform to the incisors. It is then easiest to make one side fit correctly and then to complete the other.

   - A bend should be made in the wire 2 mm from the edge of the lateral incisor at an angle such that the wire slopes backwards towards the canine.

   - A coil can now be made in this section slightly in front of and above the gingival margin of the canine.

2. Slide on the bevelled tube and fit the sleeved wire into the palate as per the buccal canine retractor.

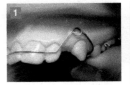
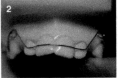

5.15 Producing baseplates

Component construction → Removable appliance construction → Fixed appliance construction

The acrylic baseplate forms the bulk of the appliance and supports all the wire components that are embedded within it. The baseplate provides anchorage by acting against the mucosa and the teeth that are not being moved. Modifications to the baseplate allow the movement of teeth, prevent tooth movement or induce tooth movement.

You will need:

- Spray-on cold-cure resin powder
- Spray-on cold-cure resin liquid
- Sodium alginate separator
- Small paintbrush
- Hydroflask
- Tungsten bur for trimming acrylic
- Polishing lathe
- Pumice
- High gloss polishing compound

Work safety

- Self-curing acrylic resin: Mix in a fume cupboard, wear gloves and wash your hands after use.
- Grinding acrylic resin: Wear eye protection and facemask, and use dust extraction.

Basic procedure

1. Cover the plaster model with separator and ensure that it has not collected underneath the wire components – this prevents acrylic flowing around the wires.

2. Add 0.5 mm of powdered acrylic from a plastic bottle to cover one-third of the palate, using a sweeping motion to create an even layer.

3. Drip on the liquid monomer slowly, adding just enough to saturate the powder. Excess liquid will cause the mass to 'puddle' in the deepest part of the palate.

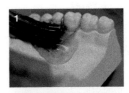
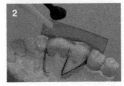
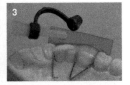

Continued over

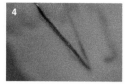
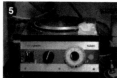
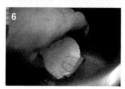

4. Repeat the powder and liquid procedure until an adequate thickness (2 mm) of acrylic has been achieved over the wires. Ensure that the acrylic is smooth and of even thickness over the whole of the appliance.

5. Place the model in a hydroflask containing hot water (55°C) and close with a pressure of 2–4 bar; leave for 15 minutes.

6. Remove the hardened appliance from the model, taking care not to break the teeth; the appliance can be flushed with boiling water to remove any wax.

7. Trim and polish.

Hints and tips

Once the baseplate has been 'sprayed on', it is best not to trim any excess as this can lift up the baseplate and compromise the fit.

5.16 Producing biteplanes

Flat anterior biteplanes

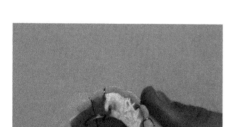

Figure 5.16.1

Flat anterior biteplanes (FABPs) are added to appliances to make sure that the posterior teeth remain out of occlusion. The clinician will specify the height and extent of the desired biteplane (FABPs are usually a half-moon shape; Figure 5.16.1). Therefore, when 'spraying on' the appliance, make sure that the anterior part is thickened by more than the specified amount so that there is plenty to trim and to bring to a high polish without the need to add any further acrylic.

Inclined anterior biteplanes

Inclined anterior biteplanes (IABPs) are very similar to the FABPs, except that the surface against which the lower anterior teeth come into contact with is inclined (Figure 5.16.2) to encourage them to procline.

Posterior biteplanes

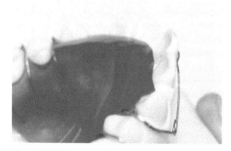

Figure 5.16.2

Strips of wax are added to the buccal surface of the posterior teeth to just higher than the desired thickness of the posterior biteplanes to allow for trimming and polishing.

Posterior bite planes (or gags) are used to keep the anterior teeth out of contact when the patient bites. This is done so that a tooth that is being moved over the bite can travel to its new position unhindered by the opposing dentition.

Component construction → Removable appliance construction → Fixed appliance construction

5.17 Extra-oral anchorage

Extra-oral anchorage is provided by headgear and can be achieved in two different ways: either a series of straps that are all connected to form a cap that fits on the head, or a neck strap. However, the use of a neck strap is not recommended for use with removable appliances.

Headgear may form the only way in which sufficient anchorage can be obtained or it can be used to add to the anchorage already in place.

Headgears are attached to the appliances via detachable facebows, which are almost exclusively bought from a dental supplier (Figure 5.17.1).

Owing to safety problems with the use of facebows (they have been known to become detached and injure the eye), it is rare to make one from scratch.

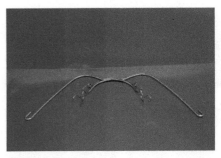

Figure 5.17.1

5.18 Functional appliance design

Functional appliances are generally used to correct skeletal discrepancies prior to undertaking fixed appliance therapy.

Using a functional appliance may reduce the length of time that a patient has to wear fixed appliances and may also reduce the need for extractions of teeth to provide enough space for the dentition.

5.19 Producing an Andresen appliance

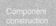

Component construction | Removable appliance construction | Fixed appliance construction

The Andresen appliance or activator is an appliance intended to function as a passive transmitter and sometimes stimulator of the forces of the perioral muscles. It is one of the activator-type appliances that induce or direct oral forces to contribute to improved tooth position and jaw relationship (Figure 5.19.1).

Andresen and other activator-type appliances are made from heat-cured acrylic, as it is stronger and easier to polish the appliance.

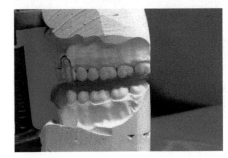

Figure 5.19.1

You will need:

- Adams pliers
- Spring-forming pliers
- Wire cutters
- 0.9 mm stainless steel wire
- 2B pencil
- Modelling wax
- Ash No. 5 carver
- Bunsen burner
- Simple hinge articulator
- Plaster of Paris
- Heat-cured acrylic
- Flask for heat curing
- Bench press
- Flask clamp
- Heat-curing water bath

Work safety

- Heat-curing acrylic resin: Mix in a fume cupboard, wear gloves and wash your hands after use.
- Grinding acrylic resin: Wear eye protection and facemask, and use dust extraction.

Basic procedure

1. Secure the models to the wax bite.

2. Articulate the models back to front such that the inside of the appliance can be easily accessed.

Continued over

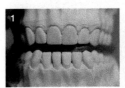
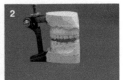

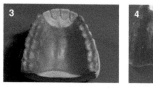

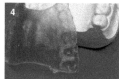

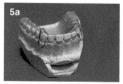

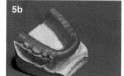

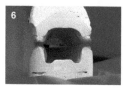

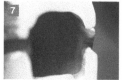

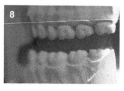

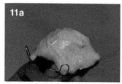

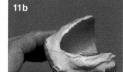

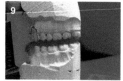

3. Wet the models to prevent the wax from sticking. Adapt a softened sheet of wax to both upper and lower models.

4. Ensure that the wax has a definite imprint in it of the teeth and mucosa.

5. Produce a labial bow on the upper model with the wire fitting high over the canine. This allows the wire to pass between the upper and lower arches when the appliance is finished. Apply a further layer of wax to the bases, bulking the base with wax anteriorly.

6. With the wax bases in place, seal the upper and lower models together.

7. Smooth the inner surface such that there is no discernable junction between the upper and lower wax bases.

8. Seal and smooth the junction on the buccal edge.

9. Trim the wax to the required size and shape, and then smooth and finish by lightly flaming the surface.

10. Place the whole set-up in a bowl of cold water. When cool, remove the waxed-up appliance from the articulated models.

11. Mix a small amount of plaster and cover the fitting surface of the wax appliance and leave to set.

12. Flask the appliance making sure that the anterior part of the appliance is pushed into the flasking plaster, and the inner surface is angled upwards. This ensures that the flask can be opened easily.

13. Flask and pack as usual.

5.20 Twin-block appliance

The twin-block appliance differs from other functional appliances in that it has separate upper and lower components. It may be considered as two appliances that work together as one (Figure 5.20.1).

The biteplanes of the two appliances meet at a 70° angle to posture the mandible forward into an ideal Class I position.

The twin-block is mainly used to treat Class II division 1 and Class II division 2 malocclusions, although the appliance can be used for a wide range of other malocclusions.

This appliance is comfortable and well tolerated. Because it is in two parts, the appliance is to be worn 24 hours a day bringing about swift completion of the treatment.

There are many variations of the twin-block appliance and for the full range it is worthwhile looking at William Clark's book *Twin Block Functional Therapy* (second edition, Elsevier Mosby, Edinburgh, 2002, ISBN 0 7234 2120 X). The appliance described here is the standard twin-block.

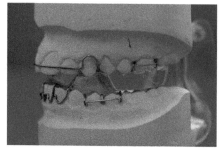

Figure 5.20.1

You will need:

- Adams pliers
- Spring-forming pliers
- Wire cutters
- 0.7 mm stainless steel wire
- Pre-formed ball-ended clasps
- 2B pencil
- Wax knife
- Modelling wax
- Ash No. 5 carver
- Bunsen burner
- Simple hinge articulator
- Plaster of Paris
- Plaster mixing bowl, spatula and knife
- Brush
- Copper-headed hammer
- Plaster saw
- Denture-processing flasks and clamp
- Vaseline
- Plaster-separating solution
- Boiling water
- Heat-curing acrylic resin
- Water or dry heat acrylic resin processing bath

Work safety

- Heat-curing acrylic resin: Mix in a fume cupboard, wear gloves and wash your hands after use.
- Grinding acrylic resin: Wear eye protection and facemask, and use dust extraction.

Basic procedure

1. Articulate the models on a simple hinge articulator, using the wax bite provided (see Section 1.17). The completed appliance aids in the location of the components.

2. Produce Adams clasps for the upper first molars and double Adams clasps for the lower premolars.

3. Make a Hawley arch (see Section 5.21) for the upper teeth to emerge from the distal of the canines.

4. Fit ball-ended clasps between the lower premolars.

5. Produce 'C' type clasps to fit the lower incisors.

6. Incorporate a midline screw into the upper arch if required.

7. For twin-block appliances it is preferable to use heat-cured acrylic for its higher strength compared with that of cold-cured acrylic. The appliance should therefore be 'waxed-up' ensuring that the upper and lower biteplanes meet at an angle of 70°. The upper should have full coverage of the premolars and molars.

8. Once 'waxed-up', the upper and lower appliances can now be flasked, packed and cured using clear heat-cured acrylic resin (for guidance, see Section 2.8).

9. Trim and polish the acrylic, taking care to preserve the biteplane where it meets the upper dentition.

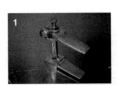
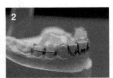
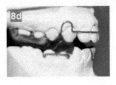
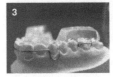
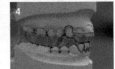
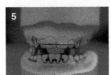
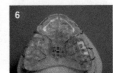
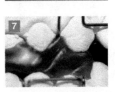
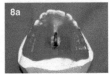
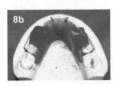
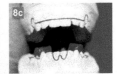

5.21 Fixed orthodontic appliances

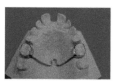

Figure 5.21.1

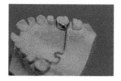

Figure 5.21.2

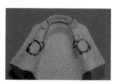

Figure 5.21.3

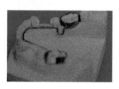

Figure 5.21.4

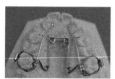

Figure 5.21.5

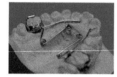

Figure 5.21.6

Trans-palatal arch

The trans-palatal arch (TPA) is made from 0.9 mm stainless steel wire that crosses the palate with a 'U' loop from the first permanent molar one side to the first permanent molar on the other. It is used to maintain arch width and aid molar movement (Figures 5.21.1 and 5.21.2).

Lower lingual arch

The lower lingual arch fulfils the same purpose in the lower arch as the TPA in the upper. It fits around the lingual mucosal wall with 'U' loops just in front of the first permanent molars (Figures 5.21.3 and 5.21.4).

Quad-helix

A quad-helix attaches to bands on the upper first permanent molars. It has four coils (helices, hence its name) that, when activated, can widen the upper arch to make room for crowded teeth or help to correct a posterior crossbite (Figures 5.21.5 and 5.21.6).

Work safety

Safety glasses should be worn and care taken when using molten solder and hot metal. Use a facemask when polishing.

You will need:

- Adams pliers
- Spring-forming pliers
- Wire cutters
- 0.9 mm stainless steel wire
- 2B pencil
- Spot welder
- Rosehead bur
- Flux
- Solder
- Soldering torch
- Bowl of water
- Rubber wheels for polishing
- Ash No. 5 carver
- Bunsen burner

Overview of basic procedure

(1) When bending the wire it may be prudent to coat the palate or lingual surface with a thin covering of wax to prevent the wire from impinging on the mucosa.

(2) The use of wax will mean that the wire will be the required distance from the mucosa.

5.22 Retainer appliance design

Following orthodontic treatment the teeth need to be held or 'retained' in their new position to prevent any unwanted relapse of the teeth. Retainers are worn for as long as possible 24 hours a day and eventually only at night.

Hawley retainers

A Hawley retainer is a simple appliance consisting of Adams clasps on the first permanent molars and a labial bow to extend from the distal of one canine to the distal of the other (Figures 5.22.1–5.22.3).

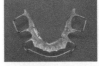

Figure 5.22.1

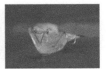

Figure 5.22.2

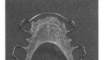

Figure 5.22.3

You will need:

- Adams pliers
- Spring-forming pliers
- Wire cutters
- 0.7 mm stainless steel wire
- 2B pencil
- Wax knife
- Modelling wax
- Ash No. 5 carver
- Bunsen burner
- Cold-cure acrylic
- Hydroflask

Work safety

Safety glasses should be worn. Use a facemask when polishing.

Basic procedure

Looking at Figures 5.22.1–5.22.3 do the following:

1. Produce Adams clasps as previously described in Section 5.7.

2. Produce a labial bow by adapting 0.7 mm wire in a smooth arch from halfway across one canine to halfway across the other; at this point make a right-angled bend towards the sulcus followed by a 'U' loop to finish at the distal edge of the canine.

3. The wire is then adapted to fit closely to the distal embrasure of the canine and the next standing tooth (this may be either a first or a second premolar depending on whether any teeth have been extracted).

4. Pass the wire directly between the two teeth on the palatal side and finish 10–15 mm into the palate with an 'L' shape at the end. Ensure the wire does not lie flat to the palate but that there is a gap of about 0.5–0.7 mm between the wire and the model.

5. To finish, produce a baseplate as previously described in Section 5.15.

Thermoformed retainers (Essix-type)

Essix retainers are popular as they are more comfortable and aesthetic than Hawley retainers and they are usually worn only at night. They are also quick and easy to make.

The design may cover all of the teeth in the arch that are to be retained or just from canine to canine. The latter design is justified in that if these teeth are held in place the rest of the arch will remain stable due to the 'keystone'-like effect of the six anterior teeth in the arch being held firm (Figure 5.22.4).

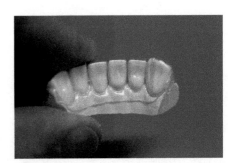

Figure 5.22.4

You will need:

- Dental stone
- Thermoforming machine
- Retainer material
- Wax knife
- Bunsen burner
- Polishing discs

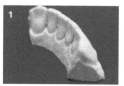
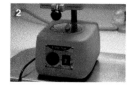
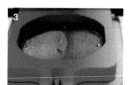
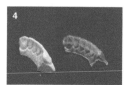
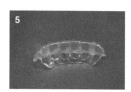

Basic procedure

1. Cast the model to the extent of the appliance required and trim the model to be as small as possible with a flat base.

2. Thermoform the material onto the model.

3. Remove from the machine and cut the excess material away using a hot wax knife whilst the retainer is still on the model.

4. Remove the retainer from the model.

5. Polish the periphery to remove any sharp edges.

Hints and tips

By making the model small, several appliances may be produced from one sheet of material.

Removable appliance construction fixed → Appliance construction → Appliance repairs

5.23 Repair and modification of orthodontic appliances

Both damaged wires and baseplates may be repaired.

Baseplate repair

You will need:

- Tungsten carbide bur
- Cold-cure acrylic
- Hydroflask
- Pumice
- Polishing compound

Basic procedure

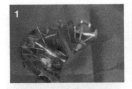
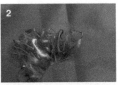
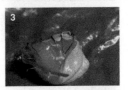
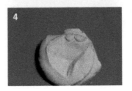

1. Clean the appliance pieces and ensure that you can fit them back together accurately.

2. If you have a model for the appliance, go to step 5; otherwise, stick the pieces of the appliance together with sticky wax.

3. Prepare a dental stone mix. Locate the appliance into a mound of die stone to make a temporary model, being careful to avoid air bubbles on the fitting surface.

4. Remove the appliance from the model.

5. Using a tungsten carbide bur trim the fractured area until all the fracture surfaces are removed. When relocated onto the model, the gap should be at least 3 mm.

6. Coat the model with sodium alginate separating solution.

7. Fit the appliance parts to the model.

8. Add acrylic as previously described in Section 5.15, and place in the hydroflask until cured.

9. Trim and polish the repaired area and polish the rest of the appliance.

Soldered repair

Wire breaks can be repaired by soldering.

You will need:

- Solder
- Flux
- Soldering torch
- Rubber wheel for polishing
- Mandrel mop for polishing

Work safety

Safety glasses should be worn and care taken when using molten solder and hot metal. Use a facemask when polishing.

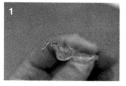
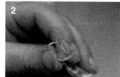
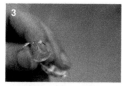
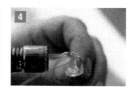
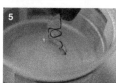

Basic procedure

1. Clean the appliance.

2. Put the two halves of the fractured wire together.

3. Fill the (in this example) arrowhead with flux.

4. Heat with the soldering torch and then add the solder.

5. Cool in water and polish to a high shine.

Hints and tips

It is advisable to not repair a wire in this way if the fracture is near the acrylic baseplate as it may melt.

Components can be added to the orthodontic appliance by soldering; this is usually by spot welding and then soldering the item to the bridges of the clasps.

5.24 Making tooth positioners

Introduction

Tooth positioners have been used in orthodontics for about 30 years in one form or another; the most common type currently used is made from clear, thin (about 0.5–0.8 mm) thermoformed plastic blanks in a pressure or vacuum forming machine. These offer a distinct advantage to the patient in that the fixed appliance can be de-bonded early so that any small final adjustments to the malocclusion can be made, and the tooth positioner becomes a retainer as well. Another use for a tooth positioner is to move a small number of teeth that only require small adjustments. There are a few brand names of tooth positioner on the market, but in general they all work in the same way and many dental laboratories are now adopting the technology that enables them to provide tooth positioners at relatively little cost without the need for expensive computer programs and 3D printers which are used by the large multinational firms providing 'invisible' braces.

You will need:

- Fret saw
- Bunsen burner
- Wax knife
- Heat resistant wax
- Sodium alginate
- Pressure/vacuum forming machine
- Model trimmer
- Strong scissors
- Abrasive discs
- Micromotor

Work safety

Safety glasses should be worn. Use an extraction hood when grinding and a facemask when polishing. Take care with hot surfaces during the vacuum/pressure forming process.

Basic procedure

1. Section from the model the teeth that are slightly out of position.

2. Trim the sectioned tooth bases so that they can be easily positioned in an ideal position within the model.

3. Once the teeth are in an ideal position wax it in place with the heat resistant wax.

4. Coat the model with sodium alginate and place in the pressure/vacuum forming machine to form the tooth positioner material onto the model – following the manufacturer's instructions.

5. Break the model out of the thermoformed material and cut the appliance to shape with the scissors.

6. Ensure covering all teeth to the most distal molar and extend beyond the gingival margin to a depth of 3–5 mm.

7. Round off the cut edge using an abrasive disc.

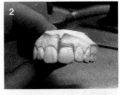
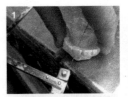
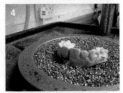
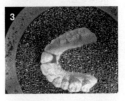
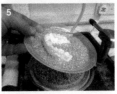
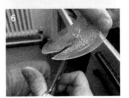
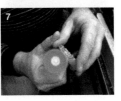

5.25 Sports Mouthguards

Introduction

The first recorded use was by the English boxer Ted 'Kid' Lewis, in 1913, who began using a 'mouthguard' made from a piece of natural rubber that had been trimmed and hollowed out so that it would fit over the maxillary dentition. He wore it to prevent chipped or broken teeth resulting from blows to the head. Modern mouthguards are now much improved, but effectively try to achieve the same goal.

It is the purpose of a mouthguard to do, quite literally, what its name implies. It should protect the teeth from fracture by an impact, protect the lips and cheeks from the teeth in the event of an impact, protect the teeth from each other when the mandible suffers an impact and also protect from bruxism (as some players tend to grind their teeth whilst participating in their chosen sport).

Dimensions of a sports mouthguard

For a sports mouthguard to be effective, it needs to cover the teeth that are most prone to trauma, so this generally means the upper incisors and canines. It must also be thick enough occlusally to ensure that if the wearer suffers an impact to the chin then the teeth do not come into traumatic contact and that the condyle is kept from traumatic contact with the glenoid fossa so that the impact energy that would pass to the base of the skull and brain is interrupted and the force dissipated.

With all this in mind, the best mouthguard should have the following dimensions:

- Anterior region, canine to canine – 5 mm (minimum)

- Occlusal region, first premolar to the most posterior molar – 5 mm (minimum).

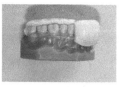

Figure 5.25.1

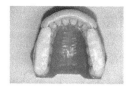

Figure 5.25.2

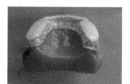

Figure 5.25.3

Elsewhere, the mouthguard can be kept to a minimum to ensure comfort for the wearer, so palatally the mouthguard should be thin and only extend by 2–3 mm beyond the teeth. This can also be repeated buccally in the premolar and molar regions.

See Figures 5.25.1–5.25.3 for buccal, occlusal and posterior views of a typical mouthguard.

You will need:

- Bunsen burner
- Wax knife
- Sodium alginate
- Pressure/vacuum forming machine
- Model trimmer
- Hot air blower
- Strong scissors
- Tungsten carbide bur
- Micromotor
- Chloroform
- Dental napkin or gauze

Work safety

Safety glasses should be worn. Use an extraction hood when using chloroform, and a facemask and extraction hood when trimming. Take care with hot surfaces during the vacuum/pressure forming process.

Overview of the typical production method for a sports mouthguard

(1) Trim the model down on a model trimmer to a horseshoe shape but keeping a good depth of model buccally and labially.

(2) Coat with sodium alginate.

(3) Place in the vacuum/pressure forming machine.

(4) Form a 3 mm blank of mouthguard material over the model.

(5) Once cool remove from the machine and trim using a clean, hot wax knife so that the material only covers the labial section (canine to canine) and the occlusal surfaces of the premolar and molar teeth.

(6) Place back in the vacuum/pressure forming machine and whilst the next 2 mm blank is heating apply hot air to the mouthguard material already formed on the model. This ensures perfect adhesion of the two materials – although they are the same material they need this extra help.

(7) Form the second layer onto the first.

(8) Once cool remove from the machine.

(9) Trim to shape with a hot wax knife.

(10) Use a tungsten carbide bur to shape and round off the periphery of the mouthguard.

(11) Finally, rub the periphery with a piece of gauze soaked in chloroform to smooth out and polish the rough surface.

Chapter 6 | OCCLUSION

6.1 Introduction to occlusion

Occlusion is the subject that is concerned with how the teeth and associated bones, joints and muscles function together.

The natural dentition

When you put your teeth together, the occlusal surfaces meet in the same position each time (Figure 6.1.1). This position is called intercuspal position (ICP) and is used extensively in dentistry. ICP is a relationship between the maxilla and mandible when the teeth are in maximum intercuspation or maximum meshing. Other terms used for ICP are centric occlusion or habit bite.

In the ICP, the occlusal load is distributed through the molars. You can feel this if you squeeze your teeth together very hard; there should be little or no pressure on your anterior teeth. The molars are well suited to distribute this load as the roots have a large surface area with which to transmit the load to the bone.

From ICP, move your mandible to the left with your teeth in contact. In most cases, you will find that the canines are the only teeth contacting or working together (Figure 6.1.2). In this excursion or movement from ICP, the left side is called the working side. The teeth on the right should not be contacting or working (Figure 6.1.3), which is why this side is termed the non-working side.

Of course, when moving your mandible to the right from ICP, you should find the right canines contact; therefore the right is now the working side and the left teeth have space between them as this is the non-working side.

In these lateral excursions, only the canines contact and take the occlusal load, whilst the other teeth are separated. The canines are better suited than the posterior teeth to distribute these sideways forces for several reasons.

- Their shape is strong enough to resist force unlike molar teeth that have fissures causing weaknesses.

- They have long roots that prevent them from moving or tipping.

- They are farther from the mandibular hinge (the temporomandibular joint (TMJ) and therefore the muscles cannot exert such high forces.

- They are also more highly innervated or sensitive than other teeth and can easily detect light contact. This stimulus informs the brain, which in turn reduces the load on the tooth. You can try this for yourself, squeeze together in ICP and feel your masseter muscle on the angle of your mandible. Now move your jaw sideways such that only the canines on one side touch and squeeze in this position. You should feel that the brain has limited the activity of the muscle.

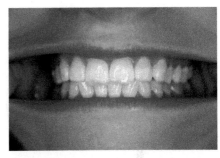

Figure 6.1.1

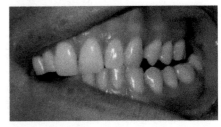

Figure 6.1.2

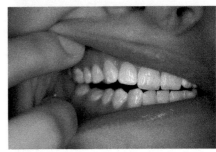

Figure 6.1.3

Basics of Dental Technology: A Step By Step Approach, Second Edition.
Tony Johnson, David G. Patrick, Christopher W. Stokes, David G. Wildgoose and Duncan J. Wood.
© 2016 John Wiley & Sons, Ltd. Published 2016 by John Wiley & Sons, Ltd.
Companion Website: www.wiley.com/go/johnson/basicsdentaltechnology

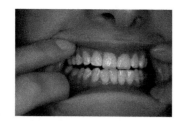

Figure 6.1.4

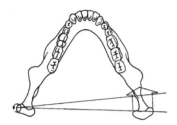

Figure 6.1.5

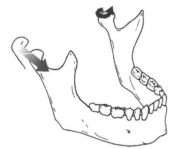

Figure 6.1.6

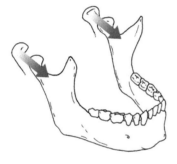

Figure 6.1.7

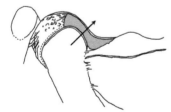

Figure 6.1.8

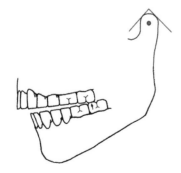

Figure 6.1.9

When the canine dictates the sideways movement of the mandible, the occlusal scheme is considered to be canine guided. This means that the canine is the only tooth guiding the sideways movement of the jaw.

The anterior teeth act in the same way during forward movements of the mandible, dictating its pathway and causing the posterior teeth to separate (Figure 6.1.4).

The two TMJs also dictate the mandibular movement at the posterior end. As the jaw moves to the left, the left or working side condyle rotates on an axis through the head as shown in Figure 6.1.5. This working side condyle may also be termed the rotating condyle.

The right side condyle moves forwards, down the articular eminence (the bony slope of the joint) and towards the left at the same time. This non-working side condylar pathway is guided by the articular eminence (Figure 6.1.6). Both condyles may translate (slide) forward in the protrusive movement of the jaw (Figure 6.1.7).

Centric relation

The mandible can be related to the maxilla in one more relationship, this time determined by the position of the condyles rather than the teeth. The condyles need to be located in their optimal position at the top of the articular eminence (Figure 6.1.8). Here, the condyles can distribute any load through the bony structures of the skull rather than using muscles to hold the condyle on the slope of the articular eminence.

When the condyles are in this position the mandible can hinge open and closed by approximately 20 mm without any forward movement. This range of movement is called centric relation (CR) and again is used extensively in dentistry. You should assume that in an ideal situation ICP coincides with the CR arc of closing; therefore, when the mandible is closed in CR, the teeth meet in ICP. This is the basic arrangement and function of the teeth in the ideal occlusion. Often, we find that this is not the case – that CR does not coincide with the maximum meshing of the teeth (ICP). The reasons for this are many and beyond the scope of this text; however, consider trying to establish all the teeth in exactly the right place and keeping them there throughout a lifetime; it will be very difficult!

When the two positions do not coincide, we use the term retruded contact position (RCP) to describe the position of the first tooth contact when the mandible is closed in CR (Figure 6.1.9).

6.2 Occlusal schemes

There are several occlusal schemes that may be easily recognised and worked with. The description above is that of the ideal occlusion, a set of four principles that were first put together in the 1920s:

(1)   ICP = RCP

(2)   Forces down the long axis of the teeth

(3)   Anterior guidance

(4)   Mutual protection.

ICP = RCP

An ICP coincident with CR is considered to be ideal as the condyles can distribute the forces generated by the muscles through bony structures. This prevents the need for antagonistic muscles to stabilise the condyle.

CR is also a reproducible position that is comfortable for the patient to use. When a new occlusion is being provided, for example when providing dentures or a full arch of restorations, the new ICP is produced to coincide with CR.

Forces down the long axis of the teeth

Cusp tip to fossa contacts result in axial forces. These forces can be distributed well by the tooth into the bone. Contact on cusp inclines result in destructive horizontal forces. These sideways forces can lead to tooth movement or fracture of a cusp.

Anterior guidance

The morphology of the canine means it can resist lateral forces, unlike the molars, which have numerous fissures that act as stress concentrators and can lead to fracture. The canine roots are long and prevent the tooth from moving or tipping. The canine and incisors are farther from the mandibular hinge (TMJ) and therefore the muscles cannot exert high forces. The anterior teeth are highly innervated (sensitive) and can easily detect forces.

Mutual protection

In ICP all teeth should be in contact – the posteriors firmly, and the anteriors lightly. Most of the force of the occlusion is carried and distributed by the posterior teeth in an axial direction; thus, the posterior teeth protect the anterior teeth.

In excursions the anterior teeth guide the movement of the mandible and cause the posterior teeth to separate. They take the load of the occlusion; thus, the anterior teeth protect the posterior teeth.

Group function

This occlusal scheme differs from the ideal occlusion in that on moving to the working side, the guidance is on two or more teeth (Figure 6.2.1). This may involve the canine. Again, this is a very workable occlusal scheme as there are no contacts on the non-working side. Producing restorations to conform to this scheme is more demanding.

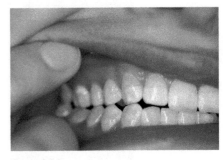

Figure 6.2.1

Gnathological occlusion

This occlusal scheme differs from the previous two in that there are contacts in excursions on both the working and the non-working sides. This situation may arise as the result of tooth wear. The scheme is not usually designed as a 'new' occlusion.

Occlusion for dentures

Dentures provide a new ICP that is coincident with CR. They are made in CR to allow optimal function (Figure 6.2.2).

Occlusion for dentures differs from that of the natural dentition, as the objective is to create a stable denture. If canine guidance was provided on the denture, the denture base would probably tip in lateral excursions.

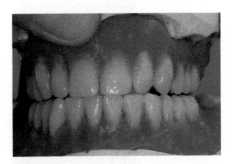

Figure 6.2.2

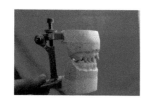

Figure 6.3.1

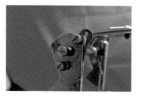

Figure 6.3.2

Figure 6.3.3

When making full dentures, the condylar pathways provide the only guidance for the mandibular movements. The denture teeth must be made to harmonise with the condylar pathways to make the dentures stable.

Each tooth is positioned such that it occludes with its opposing tooth in all excursions at all times. Therefore, in any lateral excursion both working side and non-working side are in occlusion. Here, we call the non-working side the 'balancing side'.

6.3 Articulators

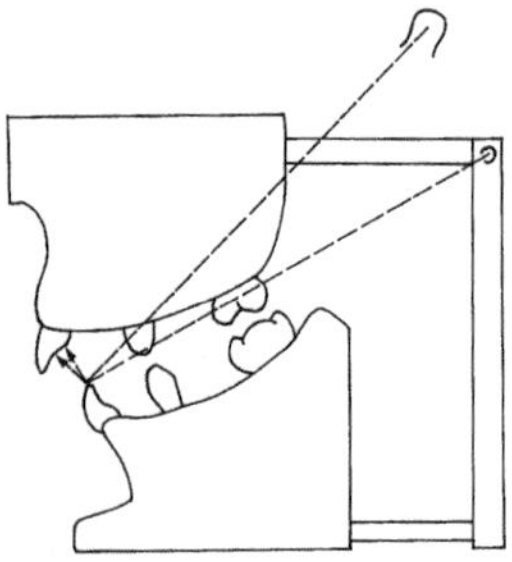

There are four categories of articulator and the type to use depends on the work being carried out. All articulators can hold models in ICP. However, due to the design of simple hinge articulators, on moving the models, they cannot accurately replicate mandibular movement (the lower and upper models will travel on a different arc from the mandible and maxilla) (Figure 6.3.1).

In Figure 6.3.2 you can see that the geometry of the articulator does not match the anatomy of the skull. The hinge is in the wrong place.

To duplicate the movement of the patient's teeth accurately, the relationship of the patient's teeth to condyle should be duplicated on the articulator. For this, the articulator must be anatomically correct.

Anatomical articulators

Figure 6.3.4

Geometrically correct articulators are required to re-create mandibular movements. This is because opening of the mandible and lateral excursions are movements around hinges (approximately). Having an anatomically correct articulator (Figure 6.3.3) allows replication of these movements.

This is also important when mounting models in CR. To take a CR record, the mandible is positioned in the hinging position with the teeth slightly apart. The record is taken and used to mount the models. To get contact between the teeth the models are then closed down on the articulator.

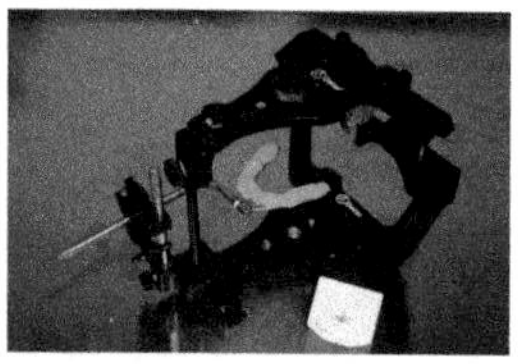

In this procedure, the mandible is opened on an arc at a fixed distance from the hinge, a CR record is taken and the models must be closed down on the articulator at the same distance from the hinge. If this distance is incorrect, errors will be introduced.

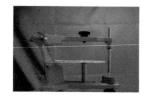

Figure 6.3.5

It is clear that the models must be positioned at the correct distance from the hinge. There are two methods, both requiring an anatomical articulator: either locate in an average position using the Bonwill triangle (Figure 6.3.4) or record the relationship using a facebow (Figure 6.3.5).

Anatomical articulators can have one of three condylar guidance arrangements:

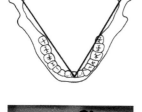

Figure 6.3.6

- Average-value (Figure 6.3.6)
- Semi-adjustable (Figure 6.3.7)
- Fully adjustable (Figure 6.3.8).

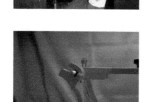

Figure 6.3.7

Average-value articulators have straight condylar paths that are set at 30°. The angle is fixed and the condylar path is straight rather than trying to re-create a true condylar pathway as shown in the diagram.

Semi-adjustable articulators again have straight condylar paths, although they are adjustable, allowing the patient's condylar angle to be measured and programmed into the articulator. Some semi-adjustable articulators also allow other variables to be adjusted, such as the distance between the two condyles, intercondylar width or the extent that the mandible can move sideways (Bennett movement).

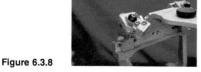
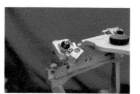

Figure 6.3.8

Fully adjustable articulators reproduce the condylar paths by recording the movements of the mandible. How the paths are recorded and mechanically duplicated determines the type of instrument. There are numerous methods: pantographic, stereographic and computerised. This type of articulator is used for precise replication of mandibular movements. This may be required when working with the more demanding occlusal schemes or for analysing the occlusion.

Articulators may also have different anterior guidance tables, and can also be considered as average-value, adjustable or custom. Most articulators are now available with a range of incisal guidance tables (Figure 6.3.9).

The condylar arrangement may also be described as:

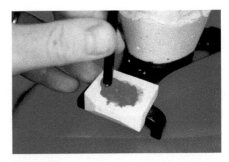

Figure 6.3.9

- Arcon (Figure 6.3.10)
- Non-arcon (Figure 6.3.11).

The term can be remembered by the words mandibul (AR CON) dyle. Thus, an arcon articulator has the condyle on the mandibular member of the articulator as in the skull (e.g. Denar). The non-arcon articulator has the condyle on the maxillary member (Condylator). For most practical purposes the difference in accuracy between the two is insignificant.

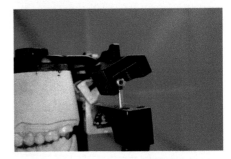

Figure 6.3.10

6.4 Facebows

There are several types of facebow, all of which allow the relationship between teeth and the condyles to be recorded and established on the articulator. The main difference between facebows is whether they record the relationship of the condyles to the mandibular or maxillary teeth. Most facebows are maxillary, recording the relationship between the maxillary teeth and condyles. This recording is used to mount the maxillary model on the articulator. Then the mandibular model is located to the maxillary model using an interocclusal record if necessary.

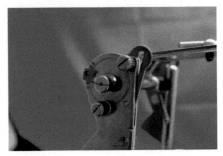

Figure 6.3.11

Mandibular facebows record the relationship between the condyles and the mandibular teeth and use this recording to mount the mandibular model on the articulator. The maxillary model is then located using an interocclusal record if necessary.

Mandibular facebows have the advantage that they allow the condylar pathways to be traced easily. This may be used to programme the condylar angle on the articulator. When using a maxillary facebow, a separate procedure is necessary to record the condylar angles.

6.5 Summary

- Simple hinge articulators can only hold models together.
- Anatomically correct articulators allow models to be moved in relation to each other.
- Semi-adjustable articulators allow the condylar angle to be adjusted.
- Fully adjustable articulators reproduce the condylar movements.
- Facebows allow correct positioning of the models.
- The Bonwill triangle gives the average position of the model.

Chapter 7 | SHADE, COLOUR AND SIZE DETERMINATION FOR DENTAL APPLIANCES

7.1 Introduction to aesthetics

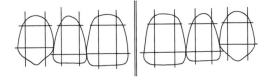

Shade taking

Colour matching or shade taking is a subjective comparison of the tooth colour to an established shade guide. Many attempts have been made to produce an objective or computerised shade analysis device with varying degrees of success. The most challenging situations are those when a single tooth requires replacement and a match must be made to the adjacent teeth. The challenge may be complicated by having discoloured, worn or restored teeth to harmonise with.

Typically, shades are taken by the clinician and sent to the technician on the prescription card. The detail required will depend upon the complexity of the case. When tackling aesthetically demanding cases it is useful for the technician to record the shade of the teeth and eliminate a possible error in communication.

Information you should find on the prescription card is as follows.

- The prescription card will typically have a diagram of the tooth. The minimum information required is a single shade which should refer to the central portion of the tooth (Figure 7.1.1).

- For more sophisticated shade taking, each square may be assessed individually. The area of translucency may also be highlighted.

- Accompanying this may be further details regarding surface finish, defects or staining. There may also be photographs and study casts to assist in communicating the shade and texture.

Figure 7.1.1

7.2 Colour terminology

Hue: This is the colour family (e.g. red, green).

Chroma: This is the saturation of the colour (e.g. increasing chroma would result from increasing droplets of dye in water).

Value: This is the relative lightness of the colour on a scale of black (low) to white (high).

7.3 Shade guides

Each manufacturer of restorative materials produces their own shade guide. You should use the shade guide that matches the materials to be used.

Basics of Dental Technology: A Step By Step Approach, Second Edition.
Tony Johnson, David G. Patrick, Christopher W. Stokes, David G. Wildgoose and Duncan J. Wood.
© 2016 John Wiley & Sons, Ltd. Published 2016 by John Wiley & Sons, Ltd.
Companion Website: www.wiley.com/go/johnson/basicsdentaltechnology

You will need:

- Colour-corrected light source
- Gloves
- Mirror
- Shade guide
- Prescription form

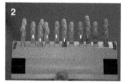
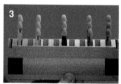

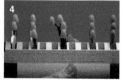
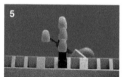

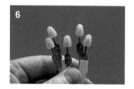

Basic procedure (using a three-dimensional (3D) shade guide)

1. Ensure the teeth are wet. If the procedure is lengthy the teeth will dry out (desiccate) and lighten in colour.

2. Set up the shade guide and check that the tabs are in the correct positions.

3. Remove all the hue shift tabs (L and R) from the shade guide and leave to one side.

4. Select the best value group from 1 to 5 (light to dark) by quickly scanning the top shade tabs past the teeth (Here a shade tab is representing the natural teeth for clarity).

5. Working with only this group, select the closest matching chroma, concentrating on the centre of the tooth.

6. Using the L and R tabs from the corresponding group, assess if there is a yellow (L) or a red (R) hue shift from the selected chroma shade tab.

7. Record the selected shade.

Hints and tips:

- Remove any strong colours from the surrounding area as these may cause a false perception of the subtle tooth colours.
- The areas of translucency are as important as the shade when attempting to match an adjacent tooth.
- Record more than one area if dealing with a demanding situation.
- Surface texture should be assessed and recorded.
- Stains or cracks should be noted on the diagram.
- Take a digital picture with the shade tab next to the tooth.

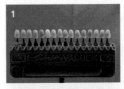
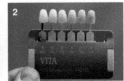
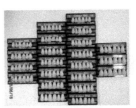

7.4 Selecting teeth for complete denture patients

This is a vital element in complete denture provision and patient satisfaction. It can ensure that the patient has 'ownership' of the dentures. It has been shown that if the patient is involved in this stage they are much more likely to be satisfied with the finished dentures. Having positive confirmation of the choice by the nurse will also make the patient happier, as they will perceive the nurse as an independent witness.

There are three basic mould shapes, round, square and tapering, to match patients with these shaped faces. Each of these has a range of sizes (Figure 7.4.1).

Whilst trying to harmonise the shape of the teeth to the shape of the patient's face (The shape of the maxillary central incisors are said to harmonise with the inverse shape of the patient's face) it can be easier to let the patient make his or her own choice, guided by the clinician and nurse. Remember, if you choose tapering teeth the contact point will be nearer the incisal edge and good appearance of the papilla/tooth relationship is more difficult to achieve.

Selecting the size of tooth can be achieved in two ways:

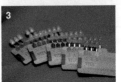

Figure 7.4.1

(1) Based on the fact that an average set of six maxillary anterior teeth measure 46 mm from distal of canine to distal of canine, a size can be chosen that reflects the patient's build, that is, >46 mm for large patients and <46 mm for smaller patients.

(2) Using a flexible ruler, measure from one corner of the mouth to the other corner of the mouth, and then use this measurement to select the appropriate size from the manufacturer's mould guide.

The manufacturer will usually recommend the appropriate size of lower anterior and posterior teeth to match your choice of maxillary teeth (Figure 7.4.2).

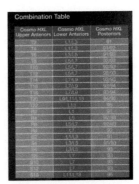

Figure 7.4.2

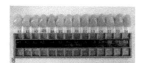

Figure 7.4.3

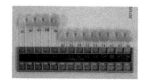

Figure 7.4.4

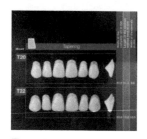

Figure 7.4.5

The easiest way to choose the most appropriate shade of tooth is as follows:

1. The hue of the teeth A–D is chosen which best harmonises with the patient's complexion (Figure 7.4.3).

2. Then, select the most appropriate value (Lightness and darkness) within the hue range, that is, A1, A2, A3, A3.5 or A4, appropriate to the patient's age (usually the older the patient's age the darker the teeth) (Figure 7.4.4).

Always remember, if the patient's wishes differ from those of the clinician and nurse, it is the patient who has to wear the dentures, so he or she should have the final decision.

Selecting teeth for partial denture patients

The selection of shade and colour of the teeth for removable partial denture cases is exactly the same as described for fixed restorations (See Section 7.3)

Determination of size and shape of tooth is made using the tooth manufacturer's mould guide, which usually has the tooth dimensions included (Figure 7.4.5).

Appendix | TOOTH MORPHOLOGY

Typical examples of maxillary tooth morphology

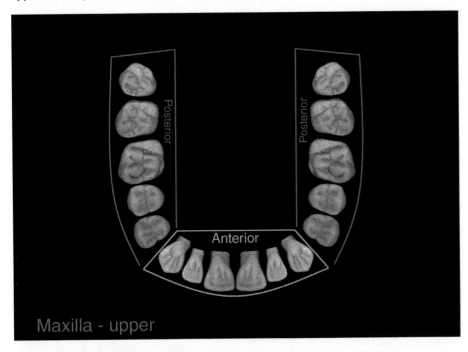

Typical examples of mandibular tooth morphology

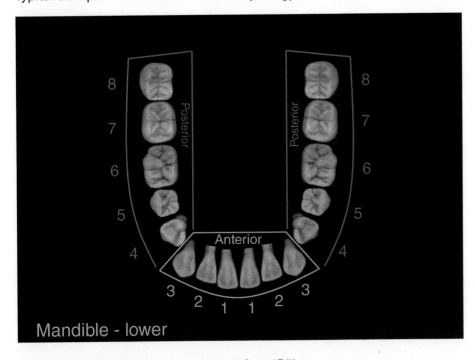

Basics of Dental Technology: A Step By Step Approach, Second Edition.
Tony Johnson, David G. Patrick, Christopher W. Stokes, David G. Wildgoose and Duncan J. Wood.
© 2016 John Wiley & Sons, Ltd. Published 2016 by John Wiley & Sons, Ltd.
Companion Website: www.wiley.com/go/johnson/basicsdentaltechnology

Typical examples of maxillary tooth morphology

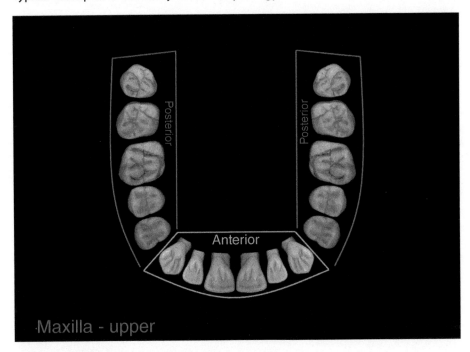

Typical examples of mandibular tooth morphology

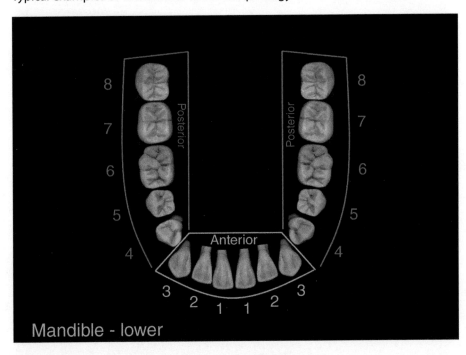

Basics of Dental Technology: A Step By Step Approach, Second Edition.
Tony Johnson, David G. Patrick, Christopher W. Stokes, David G. Wildgoose and Duncan J. Wood.
© 2016 John Wiley & Sons, Ltd. Published 2016 by John Wiley & Sons, Ltd.
Companion Website: www.wiley.com/go/johnson/basicsdentaltechnology

Glossary

A comprehensive prosthetic dentistry glossary can be found in the *Guidelines in Prosthetic and Implant Dentistry*, published by Quintessence Publishing, London, for the British Society for the Study of Prosthetic Dentistry (BSSPD).

Annealing

The process of regulated heat treatment of an alloy in order to remove work hardening strains developed during cold working, which may cause fracture.

Antero-posterior and lateral compensating curves

Downwardly convex artificial curves imposed on the occlusal plane of complete dentures. By modifying the orientation of the occlusal surfaces and so changing the effective cusp angle to harmonise with the condylar or incisal guidance angles, the curves help preserve balanced articulation in forward and lateral mandibular excursions.

Balanced articulation

An arrangement of the artificial teeth whereby the dentures provide mutual stability in all successive lateral and protrusive excursions by means of bilateral interocclusal contacts.

Balanced occlusion

A position of static denture occlusion in which the dentures provide mutual stability by means of bilateral interocclusal contacts.

Bennett shift

A lateral movement undergone by the 'rotating' condyle during lateral excursions of the mandible. It has immediate and progressive components and may be recorded by means of a pantographic facebow.

Condylar guidance angle

The sagittal angle between the Frankfort plane (or other suitable plane) and the path of the head of the condyle as it moves in mandibular protrusion downwards and forward in the glenoid fossa.

Contact surfaces

The region on the proximal surface of a tooth or a restoration that touches the adjacent tooth.

Diastema

A naturally occurring space between the anterior teeth.

Embrasure

The space defined when adjacent surfaces flare away from one another, such as those found above and below the proximal contact area.

Emergence angle/profile

The contour of a tooth or restoration, as it relates to the adjacent gingival soft tissues.

Extra-coronal attachment

Any pre-fabricated attachment positioned outside the normal contour of the abutment tooth.

Gingival sulcus/crevice

A shallow fissure between the marginal gingival and the enamel, cementum or restoration surface.

Incisal guidance angle	The sagittal angle between the Frankfort plane (or other suitable plane) and the path taken by the tips of the mandibular incisors as they move in mandibular protrusion downwards and forward in contact with the lingual surfaces of the maxillary incisors.
Interdental papilla	A projection of the gingiva filling the space between the proximal surfaces of two teeth.
Interproximal space	A gap or space between adjacent teeth within the same arch. This is divided into the embrasure space occlusal to the contact area and the septal space, gingival to the area of contact.
Interstitial surfaces	Between the proximal surfaces of the teeth within the same arch.
Intra-coronal attachment	Any pre-fabricated attachment positioned within the normal contour of the abutment tooth.
Mandibular hinge axis	The retruded axis through which mandibular opening occurs prior to forward translation.
Margin	The outermost edge or border of a restoration
Matrix	The female part, or internal slot of a two-part attachment.
Medium/macro etch	The use of salt grains to create surface irregularities able to provide a surface for resin-bonding.
Micro etch	The use of chemical or electrolytic methods to microscopically etch the grain structure of certain alloys.
Morphological contour	The overall representation as to the original natural contour or shape of the tooth or teeth.
Occlusion	The relationship between the incising or masticatory surfaces of maxillary and mandibular teeth or restorations.
Patrix	The male intersecting part, flange or projection of a two-part attachment.
Precision attachment	An interlocking device, one component of which is fixed to an abutment and the other is integrated into the pontic.
Proximal surface	The surface of a tooth or the portion of a cavity that is nearest to the adjacent tooth; the mesial or distal surface of a tooth.
Resin-bonded bridge	A fixed dental prosthesis replacing a missing tooth and requiring only minimal preparation of the abutment tooth/teeth, and relying on a composite resin luting material for its retention.
Wing	A single, or wrap around surface retainer, used with minimum preparation resin-bonded bridges/splints.

Index

Basics of Dental Technology: A Step By Step Approach, Second Edition.
Tony Johnson, David G. Patrick, Christopher W. Stokes, David G. Wildgoose and Duncan J. Wood.
© 2016 John Wiley & Sons, Ltd. Published 2016 by John Wiley & Sons, Ltd.
Companion Website: www.wiley.com/go/johnson/basicsdentaltechnology